the Healthy Pregnancy Cookbook

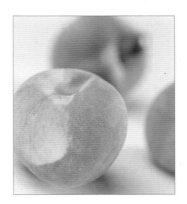

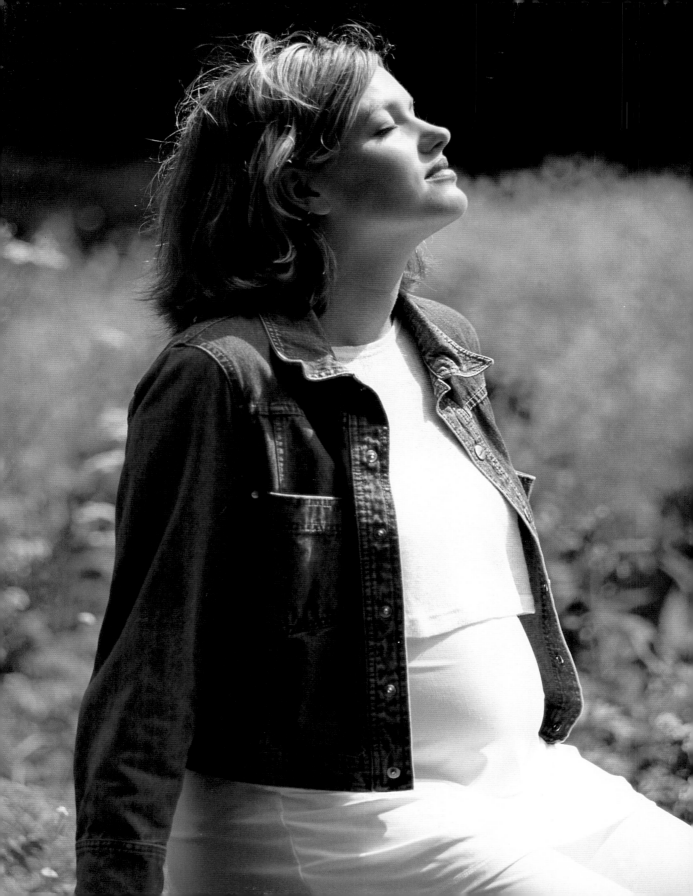

the Healthy Pregnancy Cookbook

eating twice as well
for a healthy baby

Jane Middleton
and George Rapitis

Hungry Minds™

New York, NY • Indianapolis, IN • Cleveland, OH

A QUINTET BOOK

Published by
Hungry Minds, Inc. in 2002
909 Third Avenue
New York, NY 10022
www.hungryminds.com

For general information on Hungry Minds' products and services, please contact
our Customer Care Department within the U.S. at 800-762-2974, outside the U.S.
at 317-572-3993 or fax 317-572-4002.

For sales inquiries and reseller information, including discounts, premium and
bulk quantity sales, and foreign-language translations, please contact our
Customer Care Department at 800-434-3422, fax 317-572-4002, or write to
Hungry Minds, Inc., Attn: Customer Care Department,
10475 Crosspoint Boulevard, Indianapolis, IN 46256.

ISBN   0-7645-6639-3

Contact the Library of Congress for complete Cataloging-in-Publication Data.

This book was designed and produced by
Quintet Publishing Limited
6 Blundell Street
London N7 9BH

Managing Editor: Diana Steedman
Text editor: Anna Bennett
Nutritional analysis: Jane Griffin
Art Director: Sharanjit Dhol
Designer: Isobel Gillan
Photography: Tim Ferguson Hill
Food stylist: Jacqueline Bellefontaine

Creative Director: Richard Dewing
Publisher: Oliver Salzmann

First Edition

10 9 8 7 6 5 4 3 2 1

Manufactured in China by Regent Publishing Services Ltd
Printed in China by Leefung-Asco Printers Trading Ltd

PICTURE CREDITS

Page 2: Bubbles/Frans Rombout; pages 5, 6, 21, 26, cover: Adrian Weinbrecht/ Practical
Parenting/ IPC Syndication; page 14 Rebecca Lacey/Practical Parenting/IPC Syndication;
page 20 Pangbourne/Practical Parenting/IPC Syndication.

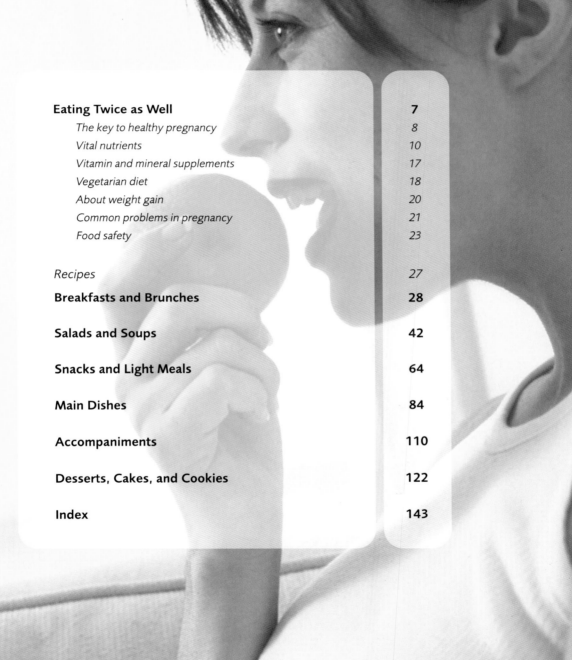

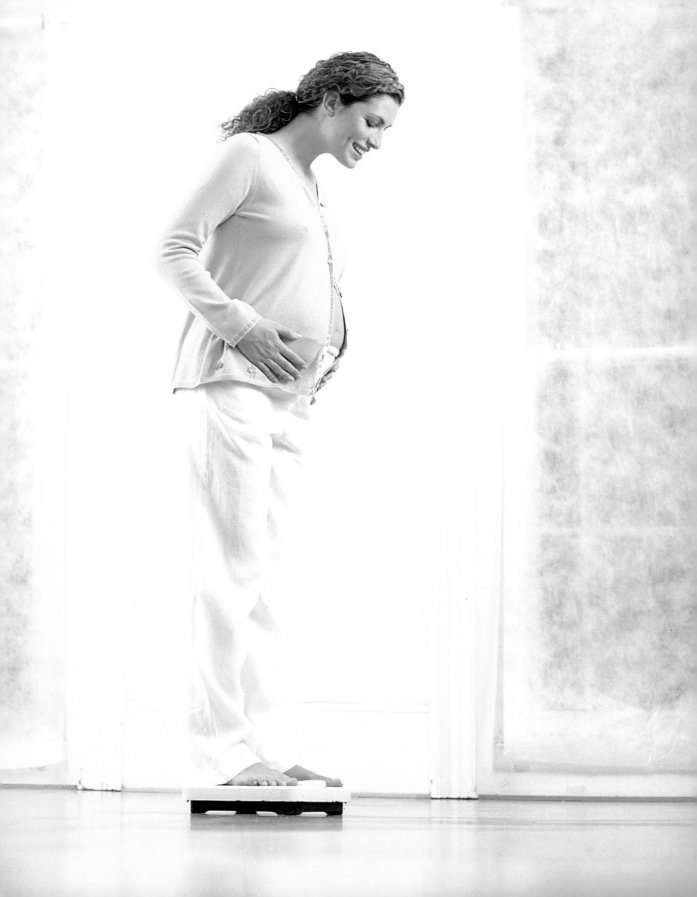

Eating twice as well

One question that, as a nutritionist, I am frequently asked by pregnant women is, "What should I be eating to ensure a healthy pregnancy?" Eating during pregnancy should above all be an enjoyable process rather than a source of worry. **You and your baby have special nutritional needs,** and eating the right foods will fulfill them. Eating the right foods will help you to produce a healthy baby, so food is very much your ally during pregnancy. While in the womb, **your baby's nourishment comes directly from your diet**. For the next nine months you are the only link your baby has to this world. Therefore, it is very important that you receive the necessary nutrients to aid in the proper development of your baby. When you eat a variety of healthy foods, you and your baby receive the energy, protein, vitamins, and minerals you both need for good health.

Several foods have a particularly beneficial effect on your baby's development. Green, leafy vegetables that contain folate, such as spinach, asparagus, and broccoli, have been shown to protect your baby significantly. Other foods such as lean meats, whole grains, oranges, tomatoes, beans, and pasta all fit excellently into a nutritious, balanced eating plan. Studies show that eating nutritious meals will help to ensure that your baby will be born at a healthy birth weight.

The introductory section of the book will show you what foods to eat plenty of, what foods you should consume in moderation, and what foods you should limit or avoid. Remember that whatever you eat, your baby eats as well!

The key to healthy pregnancy

A general guide for all healthy individuals seeking to follow a nutritious diet is the Food Guide Pyramid on the opposite page. It is derived from the United States Department of Agriculture Food Guide Pyramid, and it makes healthy eating easier to understand by showing types and proportions of foods needed in a daily balanced diet. Pregnant or breastfeeding women can use it as a guide to which foods to eat and how much to eat from each food group. Following it daily takes a little planning, so it is a good idea to appreciate how it works.

The base of the Food Guide Pyramid indicates a recommended six to 11 servings daily of grain products such as bread, cereal, rice, and pasta. Some pregnant women may think this is too much, but consider, for example, that one slice of bread counts as one serving, then a sandwich for lunch equals two servings. A small bowl of cereal and one slice of toast for breakfast counts as two more servings. And if you have a cup of rice or pasta at dinner, that's two more servings. For each day's nourishment, it is best to have the highest proportion of your servings from the base of the Pyramid.

Next in importance, and the next largest section of the Food Guide Pyramid, are three to five servings each day of your favorite vegetables, and two to four servings per day of fruits. These two groups add color, taste, and texture to your food and provide important amounts of vitamins, minerals, and fiber.

Milk and milk products, meats, and vegetarian protein foods take up a smaller layer on the Pyramid because you need fewer servings of these (two to three servings per day) than of grain products, vegetables, and fruits. Nutritionists strongly recommend that a pregnant woman consume at least three servings from the milk and milk products food group.

At the top of the Pyramid a small section depicts the contribution permitted for fats, oils, and sweets. In all the food groups, there is both naturally occurring and added fat, while sugar is added by manufacturers during food processing to foods such as ice cream, sweetened yogurt, chocolate milk, and canned or frozen fruit with heavy syrup.

Fruits, vegetables, and grain products are naturally low in fat, but many popular items, such as french-fried potatoes, and croissants, are high in fat.

This does not mean that foods like butter, salad dressings, cookies, or desserts cannot be part of a healthy diet during pregnancy. But it does indicate that these should be a much smaller part of your diet than the other food groups.

Nutritionists recommend the Food Guide Pyramid to pregnant women because it provides the best guidance to a balanced eating plan.

What counts as one serving from the Food Guide Pyramid?

Bread, Cereal, Rice, and Pasta
1 slice bread
1 ounce ready-to-eat cereal
$^1/_2$ cup cooked cereal, rice, or pasta

Vegetable
1 cup raw leafy vegetables
$^1/_2$ cup other vegetables (e.g., carrots),
    cooked or raw
$^3/_4$ cup vegetable juice

Fruit
1 medium apple, banana, or orange
$^1/_2$ cup chopped fresh, cooked, or canned fruit
$^3/_4$ cup fruit juice

Milk, Yogurt, and Cheese
1 cup milk or yogurt
$1^1/_2$ ounces natural cheese
2 ounces processed cheese

Meat, Fish, Legumes, Eggs, and Nuts
2 to 3 ounces cooked lean meat, poultry, or fish
$^1/_2$ cup cooked dry beans
1 egg
2 tablespoons peanut butter or $^1/_3$ cup nuts count as
    1 ounce meat

FOOD GUIDE PYRAMID

Daily food servings for a healthy pregnancy

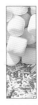

EAT SPARINGLY	**FATS AND SUGAR GROUP**	Watch out for hidden fats and anything high in sugar, such as french fries, chocolates, and canned drinks.

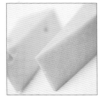

2-3 servings — **MILK, YOGURT, AND CHEESE GROUP** — **Essential nutrients** – this group includes milk, yogurt, and cheese – some of the best sources of calcium.

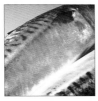

2-3 servings — **MEAT, FISH, LEGUMES, AND EGGS GROUP** — **Eat in moderation** – you should try to have some protein in every meal. Choose lean poultry and meat. Nuts and pulses are a good source of protein.

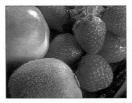

2-4 servings — **FRUIT GROUP** — **Vital nutrients** – fruit provides important amounts of vitamins, folic acid, and minerals, and are low in fat too.

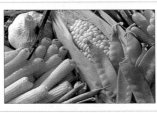

3-5 servings — **VEGETABLE GROUP** — **Vital nutrients** – vegetables add color, taste, and texture to your food and ensure you get a balance of nutrients.

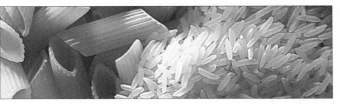

6-11 servings — **Energy sources** – whole grains, pasta, and rice are a key source of fiber and vitamins.

BREAD, CEREAL, RICE, AND PASTA GROUP

✱ Based on the USDA Food Guide Pyramid. Source: National Center for Nutrition and Dietetics

Vital nutrients

Among the nutrients that deserve special attention in the diet of pregnant women are iron, vitamin C, vitamin D, complex carbohydrates, calcium, protein, and folic acid. This section explores each one and looks at the health benefits to you and your baby.

Iron

Iron is essential for health because it makes red blood cells, supplies oxygen to cells for energy and growth, and builds bones and teeth. In other words, blood is supplying the growing fetus with oxygen which it needs in order to develop properly. Increasing iron-rich foods in your diet by eating a variety of different foods is highly recommended. The amount of iron the body can absorb from a food source varies significantly since iron availability is determined by whether it comes in the form of heme or non-heme iron. Heme iron is found in meat, fish, and poultry and is absorbed much better than non-heme, which is iron found primarily in fruits, vegetables, dried beans, nuts, and grain products. Your need for this crucial mineral doubles during pregnancy because your body must produce extra blood to support your growing baby. In addition to increasing iron-rich foods, be sure to include a vitamin C–rich food with every meal since it will help you to absorb more iron.

Vitamin C

Vitamin C (ascorbic acid) assists with wound and bone healing. It also helps the body to produce collagen, the protein that plays a part in building the body's connective tissue. Vitamin C has been shown to increase the body's resistance to infection. Both mother and fetus need this vitamin daily because it serves as a bond that holds new cells together. It helps with the growth of your baby and builds strong bones and teeth. In addition, it helps your body to absorb iron. I recommend that you include a vitamin C–rich food with every meal to get the most iron out of the other foods you eat.

Eating just one orange a day will help you come very close to fulfilling your daily requirement of vitamin C. It is best to get your vitamin C from fresh fruits and vegetables, and freshly squeezed fruit juices and smoothies.

Iron–rich foods

Excellent Sources
Pork loin chop
Lean beef (sirloin, loin, round)

Good Sources
Apricots (unsulfured)
Navy beans
Kidney beans
Pinto beans
Lentils
Spinach
Oatmeal

Useful Sources
Garbanzo beans
Beet greens
Cereal (iron-fortified)

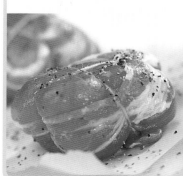
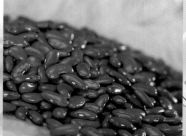
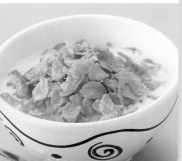

Vitamin C–rich foods

Excellent Sources
Orange
Bananas
Lima beans
Raspberries
Peas
Radishes
Broccoli
Papaya

Good Sources
Apples
Peaches
Corn
Mango
Grapefruit
Strawberries

Useful Sources
Cabbage
Tomato
Beet greens

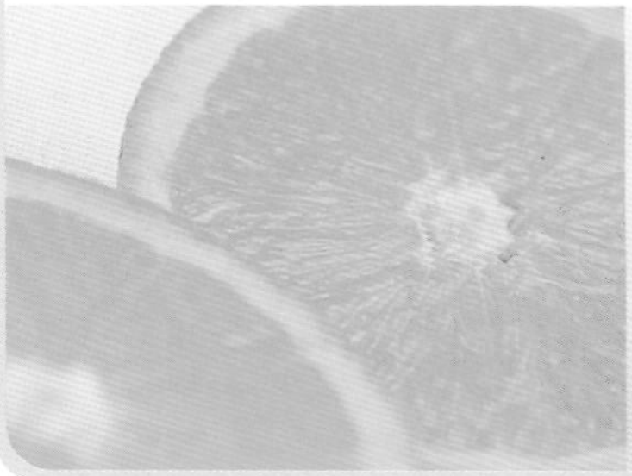

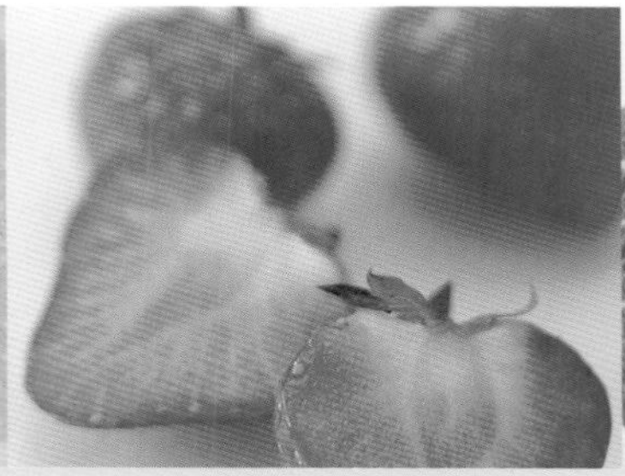

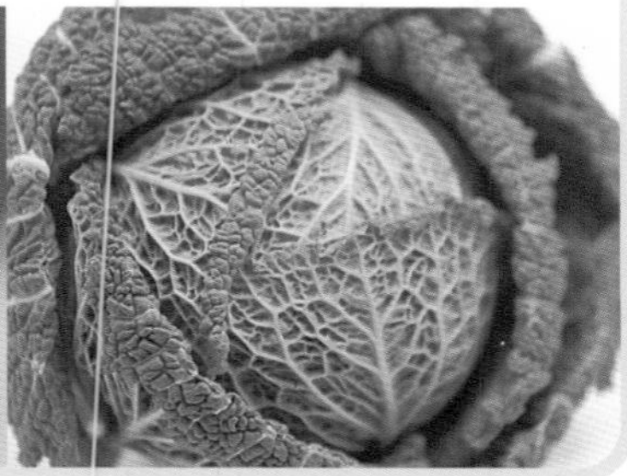

Vitamin D

Your body needs vitamin D, a fat-soluble vitamin, for growth. Its value lies in maintaining proper levels of calcium and phosphorus and helps build your baby's bones and teeth. Pregnant women need 5 to 10 micrograms of vitamin D daily, and the best sources include fish, milk, and yogurt.

The body can actually make vitamin D when it is exposed to sunlight for 10 minutes daily. This is the main source of vitamin D for most people. However, in the winter, or if you live in a region where there is less opportunity for exposure to sunlight, then you should make sure to eat a variety of vitamin D foods.

Vitamin D–rich foods

Excellent Sources
Sardines
Trout
Salmon

Good Sources
Cheese
Yogurt

Useful Sources
Egg yolks
Cereal (fortified with vitamin D)

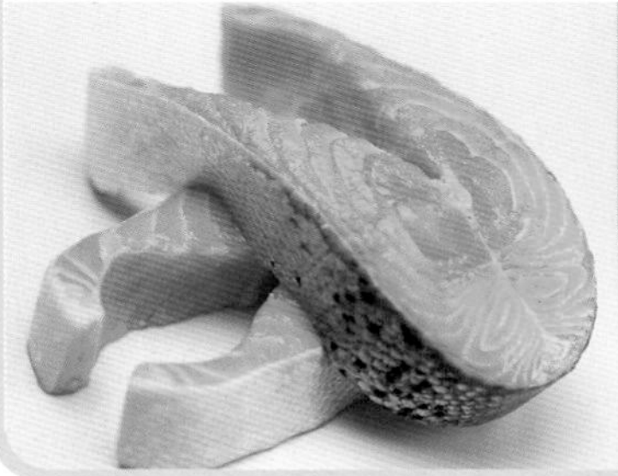

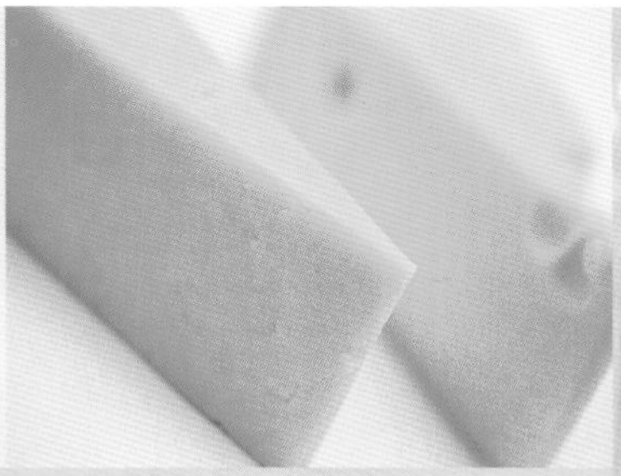

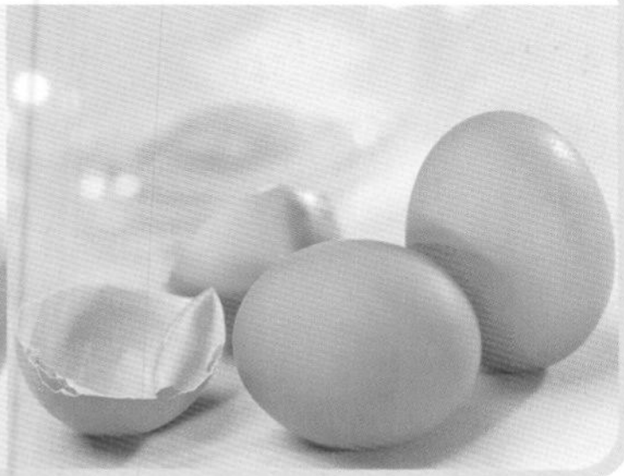

Complex carbohydrates

Whole grains (whole wheat, oats, barley, corn, brown rice) are known as complex carbohydrates, and complex carbohydrates are the body's number one fuel source. This is why they are known as a pregnancy power food. They most notably contain the B vitamins (including B1, B2, and niacin) which are needed for the release of energy from the food you eat. They also help the healthy development of the placenta, as well as other tissues in your body, by encouraging blood vessel growth. Complex carbohydrates are the base of your diet, so you should aim for at least six servings daily. Choose carbohydrates from complex sources – cereals, rice, pasta, breads, and other grains. Simple carbohydrates, like sugar and fruit, provide the same fuel, but that energy is available more quickly and lasts for a shorter time. If you feel tired or faint and need a quick boost of energy, by all means have a cookie or some chocolate, but bear in mind that an eating plan which combines the two – simple and complex carbohydrates – offers fuel, nutrition, variety, and enjoyment. One good way to combine both carbohydrates would be topping a bowl of oatmeal (a complex carbo) with apple slices (a simple carbo).

Calcium

If you take a prenatal multivitamin, it may contain very little calcium, so you should make sure to eat plenty of foods containing this mineral. The best calcium-rich foods are yogurt, milk, cheese, calcium-fortified orange juice, and tofu made with calcium salts. Your body absorbs calcium from dairy products better than it does from other food sources, so it is a good idea to increase your intake of calcium with milk and yogurt to at least three portions daily, as recommended in the Food Guide Pyramid. One cup (8 fl oz) milk or yogurt has 300 milligrams of calcium. Greens such as collards and spinach are useful sources of calcium.

Calcium is required for bone formation. You may feel that your calcium intake during pregnancy should be dramatically increased, but keep reading. In 1997, the Institute of Medicine published new dietary recommendations for calcium that were the same for pregnant and nonpregnant women: 1,000 milligrams for those aged 19 through 50 (1,300 milligrams through age 18). Based on a review of calcium research, the Institute determined that because calcium absorption actually improves during pregnancy, there was no need to recommend additional calcium.

Carbohydrate–rich foods

Excellent Sources
Oatmeal (complex)
Whole grain cereal (complex)
  with fruit topping (simple)
Barley (complex)
Bulgur (complex)
Whole-wheat bread (complex)

Good Sources
Cornbread (complex)
Plain bagel (complex)
English muffin (complex)
  with strawberry jam (simple)
Waffle (complex)
Brown rice (complex)

Useful Sources
Dinner roll (complex)
Rice (complex)
Soybeans (complex)
Raisins (simple)
Milk (simple)

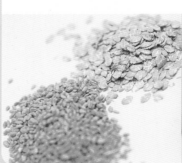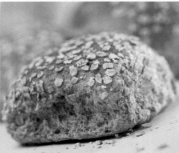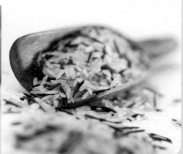

Calcium–rich foods

Excellent Sources
Milk
Yogurt
Cheddar cheese
Plain rice
Cottage cheese (calcium-fortified)

Good Sources
Canned salmon
Bread (calcium-fortified)
Orange juice
Turnip greens

Useful Sources
Collards
Spinach
Tofu

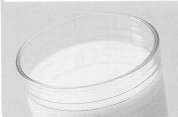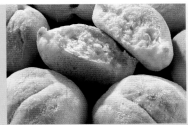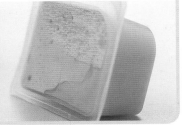

Protein

You need about 15 percent more protein in your diet when you are pregnant to provide the necessary materials for growing tissues. Excellent food sources of protein are red meat, chicken, milk, cheese, beans, lentils, and tofu. During your pregnancy, eat at least three servings of protein daily, and you will be well on your way to eating twice as well for a healthy pregnancy and baby.

What counts as one serving of protein?

Amount

1 cup cottage cheese	3 ounces cooked chicken
1 cup plain yogurt	
1 1/2 ounces cheese	3 ounces cooked lamb
1 egg	3 ounces cooked pork
1 cup tofu	3 ounces cooked fish

Folic acid

The vitamin folic acid is important in helping to prevent birth defects. It is also known as folacin or folate and can be found in some enriched foods and vitamin supplements. Studies have shown that women who consumed the recommended amount of folic acid before conception and until the twelfth week of their pregnancy reduced the risk of neural tube defects significantly. Some studies claim up to 70 percent reduction. Neural tube defects include spina bifida and brain malformations that develop within the first four weeks following conception. Folic acid intake is crucial for the health of your baby because of the protection it affords.

Natural sources of folic acid include green leafy vegetables, nuts, beans, and citrus fruits. It is actually a B vitamin, which is needed for cell division in a developing baby, and it is important in aiding your baby's development. If you were unaware you were pregnant and did not consciously consume more folic acid in your diet, don't worry. Since January 1998, regulations have required all refined grain products to be fortified with folic acid. Fortified breads, rice, crackers, pasta, and other products now provide about 40 micrograms of folic acid per serving.

Cereals, such as Total and Product 19, that contain 400 micrograms folic acid per serving are the most fortified cereals available. Always consult the nutrition information panel on the cereal package to confirm the cereal you select is fortified. You can ensure you are consuming enough folic acid by eating these breakfast foods and by taking a supplement of folic acid. This is strongly recommended by most health practitioners. It is suggested that pregnant women take 400 micrograms folic acid from supplements, plus 200 micrograms from foods that are folate rich.

Folate–rich foods

Excellent Sources
Spinach
Asparagus
Green beans
Wheat germ
Papaya
Brussel sprouts
Black-eyed beans
Cereal or bread (folate fortified)

Good Sources
Broccoli
Cauliflower
Potatoes
Peas
Grapefruit

Useful Sources
Lettuce
Cabbage
Tomatoes
Oranges
Brown rice

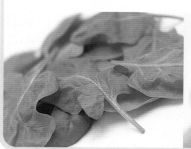
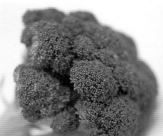
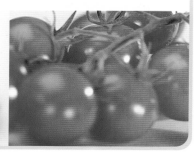

Water and fluids

During pregnancy, water and fluids play a very important role because they actually transport nutrients through your blood to your baby via the placenta. You should aim to drink at least six to eight glasses of fluids per day (3 to 4 pints), plus 1 pint for each hour of light activity. Be sure to drink an adequate amount of water each day.

A variety of fresh fruits such as oranges, canteloupe, and watermelon can also contribute to your fluid intake as well as beverages, such as cocoa or caffeine-free herbal teas and infusions. However, your consumption of caffeinated coffee, tea, colas, and alcohol should be kept to a minimum, and this is discussed in more detail on page 16.

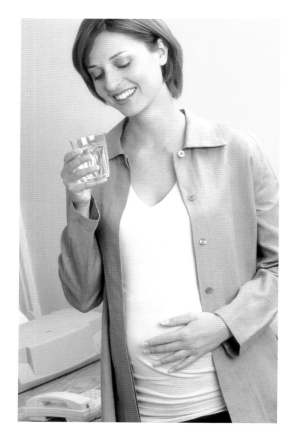

Remember to include plenty of water in your daily routine. Water helps to transport the vital nutrients you are eating to your baby.

Nutrients to take in moderation

Up to this point, we have been dealing with the key nutrients you must include in your diet when you are pregnant. The following nutrients are also important, but are needed only in moderation.

Salt

Most Americans have more than three times the recommended amount of salt in their diet. Salt is the chemical sodium chloride with iodine added, and it is sold as iodized table salt. Using salt in moderation during pregnancy is important because excessive salt intake increases the risk of high blood pressure. A pregnant woman's need for salt (sodium) in the diet is no different than that of a nonpregnant woman. However, a pregnant woman does need iodine in her diet because it helps in the development of the baby's nervous system, thyroid gland regulation, and the production of the thyroid hormone, thyroxine, which regulates metabolism. An iodine supplement is not required since a balanced diet will provide sufficient. Iodine is found in milk, probably one of the best sources, and in eggs and brewer's yeast.

Fats

Fat is good for you and your developing baby. It is needed for the development of healthy skin and vision as well as to help break down fat-soluble vitamins and essential fatty acids. It also provides a source of energy. Certain fats, such as mono-unsaturated and polyunsaturated fats, have been shown to have a favorable effect on blood cholesterol levels when eaten in moderation. These fats are usually liquid at room temperature and are found primarily in vegetable products. It is recommended you eat a combined three to four servings daily of both these fats. One tablespoon of oil (e.g., olive oil, peanut, soybean) counts as one serving of fat.

Saturated fats, such as butter and shortening, are usually solid at room temperature and are the type of fat to use in moderation. When a recipe calls for butter for sautéing, try substituting olive oil or peanut oil, both of which are monounsaturated fats.

Keep a sharp eye out for fat amounts when you are eating out, and avoid dishes that are pan-fried, crispy, creamed, fried, hollandaise, escalloped, or buttery. It is best to choose foods that have been broiled, baked, or steamed.

Foods to limit or avoid

This section covers those foods that could harm you or your growing baby.

Seafood

Many pregnant women ask "Can I safely eat seafood?" The answer is that fish is a healthful alternative to red meat during pregnancy, supplying as it does hefty amounts of the type of oils known as omega-3 fatty acids, which are needed for the development of baby's vision and nervous system as well as a healthy birth weight. It is particularly important to have these oils in late pregnancy. However, *some fish and shellfish are safer than others*. The biggest concerns about eating fish at any time, but most particularly when pregnant, are bacterial food poisoning and chemical contaminants in fish from polluted waters. Purchasing fresh fish and taking care to handle and prepare fish correctly will help reduce or kill bacteria. You have less control over chemical contaminants. Some pesticides and residues, such as PCBs and PBBs, have leached into the water supply and accumulate in some freshwater fish. With the exception of tuna, shark,

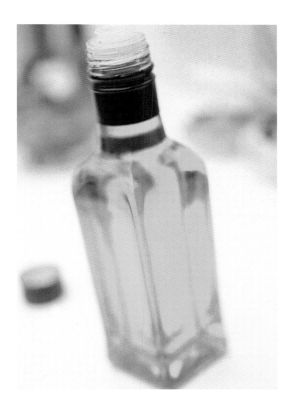

mackerel, tilefish, swordfish, and inshore species such as bluefish and striped bass, marine fish are relatively safe.

So what are your options? A general guideline is to choose low-fat fish and shellfish (e.g., orange roughy, sole, and crab) since most contaminants are stored in fatty tissue. Even though they are lower in fat, they still contain good amounts of omega-3 fatty acids.

NOTE: The above warnings have been established by the National Institute of Environmental Health Sciences, which conducts basic research on environmental health and environment-related diseases worldwide.

Raw food

Eating raw or lightly cooked meat, poultry, and eggs poses risks of salmonella poisioning to pregnant women. (See food-borne illness on page 24.)

These foods, in a raw or lightly cooked state, contain tiny microorganisms which can cross the placenta of the mother and infect the developing fetus. *Raw fish, such as sushi, should be avoided during pregnancy.* You can still have some types of sushi, but select only those that are made with cooked fish or vegetables.

You may not realize that some recipes for favorite foods, generally homemade or at restaurants, call for raw or very lightly cooked eggs. Some common recipes that call for raw eggs include homemade ice cream, homemade mayonnaise, Caesar salad dressing, eggnog, raw cookie dough, homemade hollandaise sauce, tiramisu, and chocolate mousse.

Liver

Liver contains extremely high levels of vitamin A, which has been shown to pose pregnancy risks (see Vitamin supplements, page 17). A 3-ounce serving of beef liver contains 9,000 RE (retinol equivalents). Veal liver is close behind – a 3-ounce serving contains as much as 7,000 RE. These are very high amounts when compared to the recommended daily allowance for vitamin A of 800 RE.

Although it has not been proven that eating liver causes birth defects, a study carried out in 1995 concluded that women who consumed 10,000 International Units (IU) of vitamin A daily (3,000 RE) in the first two months of pregnancy were at twice the risk of having a baby with birth defects. My advice is to play it safe and avoid liver.

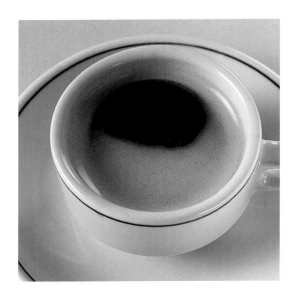

Caffeine

Studies have found no reliable evidence to link the consumption of caffeine to cancer, miscarriage, and birth defects, but since it can constrict blood vessels and increase heart rate, *doctors recommend that pregnant women switch to decaffeinated coffee* and limit their consumption of caffeinated coffee.

Don't forget that other substances contain caffeine: a 12-ounce can of cola contains almost 50 milligrams of caffeine, a cup of tea 27 milligrams, and 1 ounce of dark chocolate 20 milligrams.

Alcohol

The jury is out on light or moderate drinking during pregnancy, but most experts will advise abstinence. Many studies have shown that alcohol can harm a developing baby, so health experts recommend that pregnant women avoid alcohol altogether. According to the American College of Obstetricians and Gynecologists and the American Academy of Pediatrics, there is no safe amount of alcohol for a pregnant woman, and drinking on a regular basis can affect a developing child.

One excellent alternative to alcohol is a fruit spritzer or fruit punches. The bottom line is, before you drink alcohol, check with your doctor to see what s/he advises.

NOTE: You do not need to worry if you were a moderate drinker before you knew you were pregnant, because it is daily and binge drinking that has been shown to be harmful.

Peanuts

Peanuts, a very inexpensive source of dietary protein, are probably one of the world's most common allergenic food. Symptoms of a reaction to peanuts include flushed face, hives, difficulty in breathing or swallowing, and rapid heartbeat.

An allergic reaction during pregnancy, or indeed at any time, can be fatal, so it is important to know whether you are peanut-sensitive or not. If you do not know, visit your health practitioner to be screened, particularly if you, your baby's father, or your baby's brother or sister suffer from asthma, eczema, hayfever, or other allergies.

People who are allergic to peanuts must make sure to check food labels for less easily recognized terms such as "hydrolized vegetable protein" or "ground nuts," which both contain peanuts. They should avoid all nuts, and cold pressed peanut oil or oil contaminated with peanut protein, and thoroughly wipe down all countertops that have come in contact with peanut product. Light olive oil is the best substitute for peanut oil.

Those who know for sure they are not peanut sensitive can safely use peanut oil.

Vitamin and mineral supplements

Fruits and vegetables are packed with vitamins and minerals, so as long as you eat enough of them, you can get all the nourishment you need from food instead of relying on supplements. Many people do not realize that supplements should not be necessary in a well-balanced diet.

Many pregnant women ask if they should take a vitamin and mineral supplement or a prenatal vitamin early in pregnancy. Several studies have shown a reduced risk of a number of birth defects in babies born to women taking a multivitamin and mineral supplement before and early in pregnancy. Folic acid, for example, has been shown to be an extremely beneficial supplement.

On the other hand, studies have indicated that taking large amounts of vitamin A (over 10,000 IU per day for months at a time) and vitamin D (over 1,000 IU regularly) may cause birth defects. Usually the only way to ingest these extremely high amounts is by taking specific supplements. Vitamin A supplements should not be used routinely during pregnancy, but if they are, not more than 5,000 IU per day should be taken. Supplements of beta-carotene, a precursor of vitamin A, have not been found to cause birth defects. Most healthcare providers will recommend that you take a special pregnancy supplement that contains a safe amount of vitamin A.

Many pregnant women ask if they should take an iron supplement. The answer is that it is best for you to consult your doctor or midwife to prescribe one for you if s/he feels it is necessary. Your doctor or midwife may recommend a daily ferrous iron supplement in the second and third trimesters.

As a general rule, most prenatal vitamins should contain a greater amount of folic acid, iron, and calcium than are found in a standard multivitamin.

NOTE: Always consult your healthcare practitioner before taking any supplements.

Preserving nutrients in food

The greatest favor you can do for yourself and your baby is to prepare food in a way that provides maximum nourishment. Certain foods, such as vegetables, should be cooked correctly or they can lose their nutritive value. For example, vitamin C is easily destroyed in boiling water.

Use the following simple tips to help preserve the nutrients in your food:

- Steam vegetables or sauté them in a small amount of oil to help retain their health-giving minerals and vitamins. Using healthier cooking methods will also retain the colors of vegetables and fruit.

- Over-boiling vegetables can destroy important nutrients.

- Cook fruits and vegetables whole and unpeeled, whenever possible. Their skins contain disease-fighting agents called phytochemicals.

- Wait 30 minutes before drinking coffee or tea after a meal. Caffeine prevents the absorption of nutrients by the body.

Vegetarian diet

Many vegetarian women ask if their vegetarian diet is appropriate for a healthy pregnancy. The answer is yes, and furthermore, studies have shown that weights of infants born to well-nourished vegetarian women have been equal to birth weight norms of infants born to nonvegetarians.

Consumer demand for vegetarian options has resulted in an increasing availability of foods that offer more choice for vegetarians. A vegetarian diet that includes legumes (e.g., kidney beans, garbanzo beans), soy foods, dairy products, and eggs can supply more than enough protein and other essential nutrients. Your body needs 60 grams of protein daily during pregnancy, so obtaining adequate protein from foods such as soybeans and eggs is essential. If you eat three servings of foods containing excellent sources of protein daily, you should have no problem fulfilling your protein requirements during pregnancy.

The Vegetarian Food Guide Pyramid is derived from the United States Department of Agriculture Food Guide Pyramid. It can be used by vegetarian women as a guide to good eating for a healthy pregnancy. The chart opposite indicates the suggested servings needed daily from each of the food groups, and emphasizes a wide base of foods to be included at every meal: from fruits and vegetables to whole grains (oats, wheat, whole-wheat bread, barley, noodles, pasta, corn). The middle sections include legumes, nuts and seeds, dairy and low-fat cheese, milk (almond, dairy, rice, and soy).

The top of the Pyramid consists of vegetable fats, oils, sweets, and salt. These are foods to be eaten occasionally or in small quantities.

The diet of pregnant vegan women (i.e., those who do not eat animal or dairy products) should be supplemented with vitamin B12 daily. Be sure to consume one serving daily of a food that is fortified with vitamin B12, such as many breakfast cereals and certain brands of soymilk.

Plan a healthful vegetarian diet during your pregnancy by following these guidelines:

- Choose a variety of foods, including whole grains, vegetables, fruits, legumes, nuts, seeds, and, if desired, dairy products and eggs.

- If animal foods such as dairy products and eggs are used, choose lower-fat versions. Cheeses and other high-fat dairy foods should be used in moderation in the diet because of their saturated fat content.

What counts as one serving from the Vegetarian Food Guide Pyramid?

Grains, Cereals, and Breads
1 slice of bread
$1/2$ cup cereal
$1/2$ cup rice
$1/2$ cup pasta

Vegetables
$1/2$ cup chopped raw or cooked vegetables
1 cup raw leafy vegetables

Fruits
$3/4$ cup fruit juice
$1/4$ cup dried fruit
$1/2$ cup canned fruit
1 medium-size fruit, e.g apple, orange, banana

Milk, Yogurt, and Cheese
1 cup soymilk
1 cup yogurt
$1^1/2$ ounces cheese

Legumes, eggs, and meat substitutes
$1/2$ cup legumes
2 tablespoons nuts, seeds
1 cup tofu
1 egg
$1/4$ cup tofu
2 tablespoons peanut butter

VEGETARIAN FOOD GUIDE PYRAMID
Daily food servings for a vegetarian pregnancy

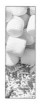

EAT SPARINGLY	FATS AND SUGAR GROUP	Butter, oils, candy, and salt.

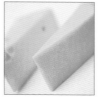

2-3 servings	MILK, YOGURT, AND CHEESE GROUP	Low-fat or non-fat milk, yogurt, and cheese.

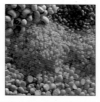

2-3 servings	LEGUMES, EGGS, AND MEAT ALTERNATIVES GROUP	Dried beans (kidney beans, navy beans, etc.), eggs, tofu, nuts, seeds, and meat alternatives.

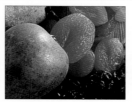

2-4 servings	FRUIT GROUP	Citrus fruits, apples, soft fruits, bananas. grapes, pineapple, and avocados.

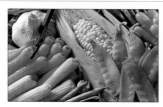

3-5 servings	VEGETABLE GROUP	Cabbage, broccoli, asparagus, bell peppers, tomatoes, roots, and potatoes.

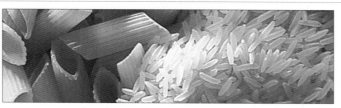

6-11 servings		Bread, oats, couscous, noodles, corn, rice, and pasta.

BREAD, CEREAL, RICE, AND PASTA GROUP

✱ Based on the USDA Food Guide Pyramid. Source: National Center for Nutrition and Dietetics

About weight gain

The range of weight gain in pregnancy varies from woman to woman. A woman who was underweight before getting pregnant may gain relatively more weight than an overweight woman. While there is no one answer to the question of correct weight gain, the best weight gain is around 20 to 30 pounds. You may be eating for two, but that doesn't mean you can double your intake.

If you are fairly active and not overweight, 200 extra calories (two slices whole-wheat bread) a day should be sufficient. For more active individuals or those of big build, your doctor may suggest up to 500 extra calories a day. Many pregnant women worry they may not lose the extra pounds they put on during pregnancy, once they deliver their baby. The chances are the pounds will come off, especially if you decide to breastfeed. Breastfeeding is not only an excellent source of nutrition for the newborn, it can help with the mother's weight loss. Producing breastmilk requires extra calories and these calories can come from the extra pounds gained during pregnancy. Most weight gain is not fat, but fluid, and because losing weight after pregnancy may be a high priority for some women, here is a breakdown of where you could expect to lose the extra weight. The fetus itself accounts for close to 7 pounds. In addition, the placenta, amniotic fluid, and some water retention could add up to another 12 pounds. Your breasts and uterus are also larger and account for about 5 more pounds together. Add this up and you have 24 pounds, which may not prove too difficult to lose while you continue to follow a healthy eating plan.

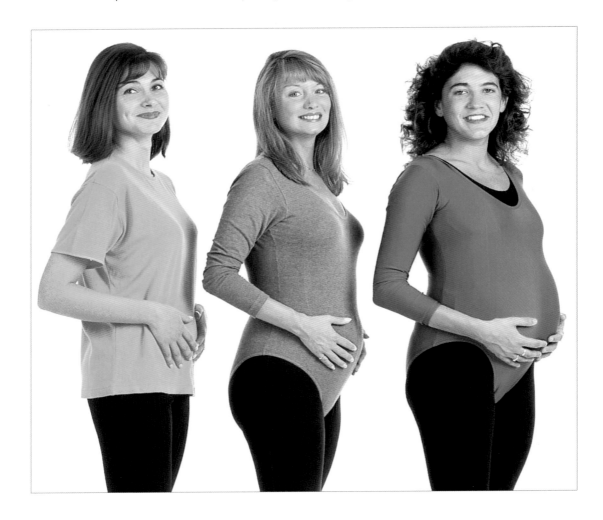

Common problems

Nausea and vomiting

Some 70 percent of women experience nausea within the first three months of pregnancy and about half experience vomiting. For some women it lasts longer. The nausea tends to be more pronounced in the mornings and can lead to vomiting (hence the term "morning sickness.") Said to be the result of physical and hormonal changes, as well as the stress of pregnancy, it can be triggered by certain odors. Remember, although you will prefer not to eat when you feel nauseous, you will be depriving your baby of important nutrients, so it is better to try to "eat through" the nausea for the health of your baby.

What can be done to lessen the effects of morning sickness? When eating seems particularly difficult, try to have several mini-meals throughout your day. Although you will not feel like eating, snacking can actually alleviate some of the nausea.

Another suggestion is to eat dry foods, such as crackers, before getting up in the morning. Foods like whole-wheat crackers and breakfast cereals can help to settle your stomach, and ready-to-eat cereals such as instant oatmeal are simple to prepare. Several of

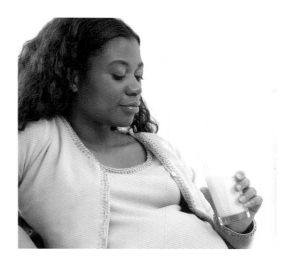

the recipes in this book are ideal for mini-meals. Keep your refrigerator stocked with yogurt, tofu, bagels, peaches, and oranges which can serve as simple meals when the nausea sets in.

Ginger can relieve nausea and morning sickness in pregnancy because it helps to promote gastrointestinal circulation. It is also a very effective remedy for heartburn.

Fresh ginger in root form can be bought from most

Foods to Combat Morning Sickness

Excellent	Good	Useful
Ginger Tea	Steamed vegetables	Hard candy
Gingerale	Soft fruits (i.e., bananas,	Lemonade
Crackers	peaches)	Potato chips
Toast	Mashed potatoes	
Plain rice (unbuttered)	Plain yogurt	
Chicken breast (skinless)		
Turkey breast (skinless)		
Plain noodles (unbuttered)		

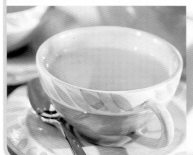
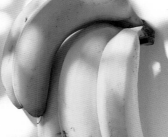
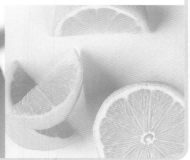

grocery stores. Use it to prepare ginger tea, and try to drink one cup a day, or prepare it as a marinade ingredient.

To make ginger tea, peel the skin and shred a teaspoon of the flesh into a small pan, add one cup of water and gently simmer for about 5 minutes. Remove from the heat, cover, and allow to steep for 5 minutes before drinking.

NOTE: If you have severe nausea or vomiting and cannot hold down food or fluid for 12 hours, consult your doctor.

Food cravings

During pregnancy you may find your taste buds crave unusual combinations of foods, perhaps even the clichéd pickle and ice cream sundae! Usually these cravings are harmless if kept under control. If you long for ice cream, for instance, and eat just one scoop, no harm is done. However, if you indulge in a gallon carton of ice cream, you are bingeing.

If at anytime you notice unusual cravings for ice, clay, or cornstarch you may be experiencing a condition called pica. Some researchers believe this is a sign of mineral deficiency, but there is no convincing evidence that it has any physiological significance.

There may be some foods you will find impossible to eat. Instead of forcing yourself, try substituting a food from the same food group. Remember, if you go a little off track with your healthy eating, you can quickly get back by following the guidelines of the Food Guide Pyramid.

Constipation and hemorrhoids

Constipation and hemorrhoids are not uncommon during pregnancy. The increased amount of hormones produced during pregnancy can slow down the digestive tract as well as put increasing pressure on your expanding uterus.

Hemorrhoids are varicose veins in and around the rectum. If you notice an increase of rectal itching accompanied with pain or blood, you may have hemorrhoids. They can be caused by constipation, which you should try to avoid. Make certain you are drinking a minimum of eight glasses of fluids daily (see page 14). You can also increase your intake of high-fiber foods such as whole grains, beans, brown rice, vegetables, and fruits with skins. Eating at least five fiber–rich food servings per day will help to prevent constipation and hemorrhoids.

Fiber-rich foods

Excellent Sources	Good Sources	Useful Sources
Cooked oats	Navy beans	Green peas
Wheat germ	Whole-wheat bread	Bread
Black beans	Brown rice	Tomatoes
Raspberries	Baked potato	Hummus
Winter squash	Green beans	
Pears		
Papaya		
Oranges		

Food safety

Organic food

It makes good sense for a pregnant woman to eat organic food for the health of her baby.

"Organic" is a labeling term that denotes production under the authority of the Organic Foods Production Act. The principal guidelines for organic production are to use materials and practices that enhance the ecological balance of natural systems. Organic food handlers, processors, and retailers adhere to standards that maintain the integrity of organic agricultural products.

The primary goal of organic agriculture is to optimize the health and productivity of interdependent communities of soil life, plants, animals, and people. Farmers must grow produce for three years without the application of synthetic pesticides or chemicals. The farm, its equipment, and any processing facilities are inspected by an independent agency unaffiliated with the grower, the processor, or the vendor, and are then issued a certificate from that agency certifying the farm's produce as "organic."

Certified organic produce is not essentially healthier than produce that has been grown under nonorganic conditions – the nutritional content of a particular vegetable does not change – and there is no scientific evidence to show that organic food is more nutritious. The lack of synthetic pesticide residues on organically grown produce, however, ensures a safer product.

Guidelines for good food safety

* Cook all meats, poultry, and seafood thoroughly. Wash raw vegetables before cooking.

* Avoid soft cheeses or mold-ripened, and blue-veined hard cheeses. Cream and cottage cheeses are safe.

* Cook leftover foods or ready-to-eat foods (like hot dogs) until steaming hot (hot dogs should be cooked to an internal temperature of 165°F).

* While the risk of listeriosis (see page 24) is low, pregnant women may choose to avoid deli meats. Thoroughly reheat cold cuts and chilled convenience foods.

* Keep salads and uncooked foods away from raw eggs, meat, and poultry.

* Maintain refrigerator temperatures at 40°F.

* Wash your hands. It is the single most effective way to prevent the spread of germs.

Food-borne illness

Listeriosis

Certain soft or mold-ripened cheeses (i.e., feta, Brie, Camembert), blue-veined hard cheeses and Mexican-style cheeses, and ready-to-eat meats (hot dogs, deli turkey, chicken, and ham) have been associated with a form of food poisoning called listeriosis. Listeriosis is caused by a bacterium (listeria monocytogenes), and is especially dangerous for pregnant women. When a pregnant woman is infected with listeriosis, she may have a miscarriage or stillbirth. Other foods that may be contaminated with listeria include undercooked meats, poultry, fish, unpasteurized milk, purchased salads, paté, quiche, or cold meat pies which will not be reheated. When food is properly cooked it poses no threat. Most people do not become ill when they eat listeria-contaminated foods. However, pregnant women are 20 times more likely than other healthy adults to get listeriosis, and more likely to become dangerously ill from it. Listeriosis often starts as an influenzalike illness with fever, muscle aches, and chills and, sometimes, nausea or diarrhea. However, it can progress to potentially life-threatening meningitis (infection of the membranes covering the brain, with symptoms such as severe headache and stiff neck). A pregnant woman should contact her doctor if she develops any of these symptoms. A blood test can be performed and may show positive. If so, the infection can be treated with antibiotics to protect the health of your baby.

Salmonella

Every year, approximately 800,000 to 4 million cases of salmonella are reported in the United States. This is a food-borne illness about which pregnant women need to be cautious. The symptoms of salmonella include cramps, vomiting, diarrhea, and fever. Contaminated foods are often of animal origin, such as beef, poultry, milk, or eggs, but all foods, including vegetables, can become contaminated. Contamination may be from the unwashed hands of an salmonella-infected person.

Raw or lightly cooked eggs are one of the top carriers of salmonella and all retail shell-egg cartons carry the warning: "To prevent illness from bacteria: keep eggs refrigerated, cook until yolks are firm, and cook foods containing eggs thoroughly."

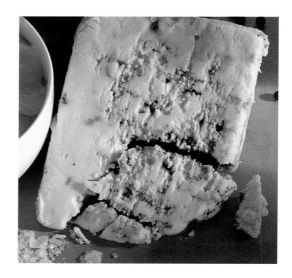

Pregnant women must avoid eating undercooked meat, chicken, and fish. Cross-contamination of foods should be avoided. Uncooked meats should be kept separate from cooked foods and ready-to-eat foods. Hands, cutting boards, counters, knives, and other utensils should be washed thoroughly before, during, and after handling uncooked foods.

Toxoplasmosis

Toxoplasmosis is an infection caused by the parasite *Toxoplasma gondii*. More than 60 million people in the United States have been exposed to the *Toxoplasma* parasite. Common sources of infection are raw or undercooked meat (particularly pork, lamb, and venison), unpasteurized milk, the feces of animals, and soil contaminated by bird or animal feces.

Toxoplasmosis affects the brain. Less commonly, toxoplasmosis can cause blindness, and can affect the lungs and other parts of the body. A healthy immune system, proper food hygiene, and special care when gardening or dealing with pets, controls the parasite and prevents illness.

Pregnant women can avoid toxoplasmosis by making sure that any meat is cooked until it is no longer pink inside; wearing gloves while gardening or working with soil or sand; and having someone else change cat litter. There is no need to give up a pet cat or dog, but avoid adopting or handling stray animals.

Eating tips for a healthy pregnancy

Here is a simple checklist to pinpoint a nutritious eating plan:

* Eat a balance of foods from all the food groups in the Food Guide Pyramid.

* Drink at least six to eight glasses of fluids daily.

* Stop alcohol consumption and smoking.

* Don't skip meals.

* Enlist the help of your partner in your healthy eating habits.

* Avoid drinking tea or coffee within 30 minutes of eating—these beverages can inhibit the absorption of nutrients, especially iron.

* Keep a food diary to check your daily requirements.

* Combat nausea and morning sickness by eating mini-meals throughout the day.

* Have any supplements prescribed by your health practitioner rather than buying them over-the-counter.

* Breastfeed your baby for nutritional and developmental benefits, and post-partum weight loss.

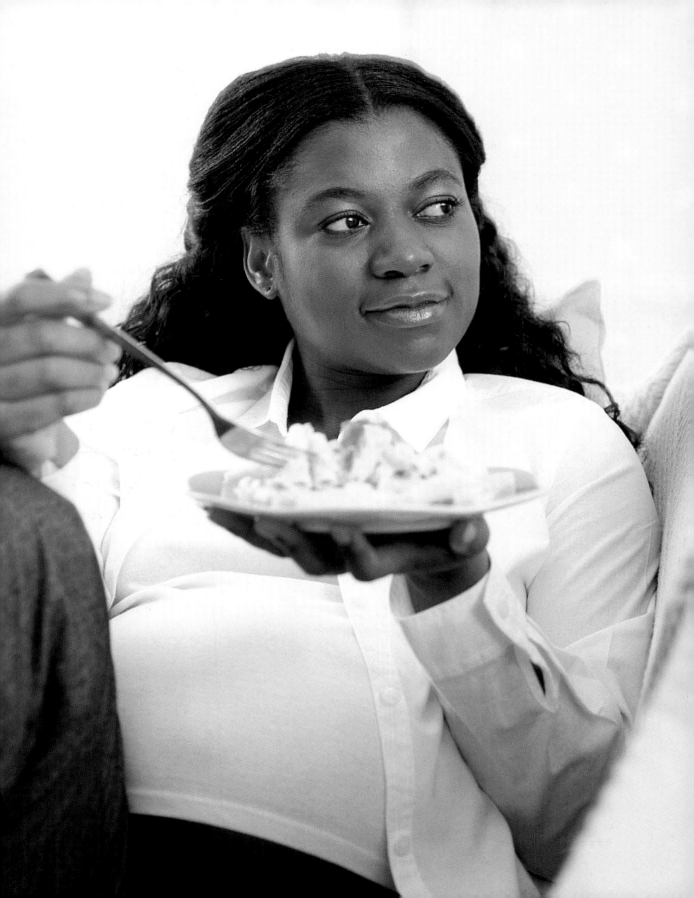

Recipes

———

Eating a balanced and healthful diet throughout your pregnancy is the goal – but sometimes there are challenges to overcome. You may be tired, you may feel nauseous, and food may taste different to you. But nonetheless, it's important to eat – and eat well – during your pregnancy and the recipes in this book are designed to help you do that.

One of the great things about pregnancy is that it gives us a chance to re-evaluate our relationship with food. Many women today spend a great deal of time worrying about dieting. Now that you're pregnant, forget about actively dieting. Instead, concentrate on seeking out good, wholesome food, eat according to your appetite, and try to nourish yourself fully. If you do this, you will be better equipped to handle the rigors of pregnancy and labor and your baby will benefit too.

The recipes were chosen primarily to help you enjoy good food during your pregnancy. They rely on fresh ingredients, simply prepared, and are rich in the essential nutrients discussed on pages 7 to 25. But eating isn't just about the pursuit of nutrients in order to be more healthy. Eating is also about pleasure. Food can raise your spirits, offer comfort, and pick you up when your energy levels are low. At a time when your appetite is affected by your mood more than ever before, this book aims to provide you with recipes that you will feel like eating: comfort foods, such as soothing pastas, creamy soups, and childhood favorites; spicy dishes for when your taste buds crave stimulation; fresh, vibrant salads and juices to perk you up; and hearty casseroles for when you feel hungry all the time.

———

A note on ingredients

Read labels carefully so you can be fully informed about the food you are buying. Given the choice between, say, plain yogurt sweetened with a little honey or maple syrup, and a flavored yogurt containing artificial sweeteners and other additives, it is clear that the first one is the healthier product. I would particularly recommend buying organic eggs and locally produced fruit and vegetables whenever these are available.

A note on nutritional guidance

Values are given per serving for the main nutrients, while the vitamins and minerals that are important for pregnant women are categorized to indicate either: excellent values = ✔✔, or good values = ✔. Ingredients that are optional have not been included in the analysis.

Breakfasts
and Brunches

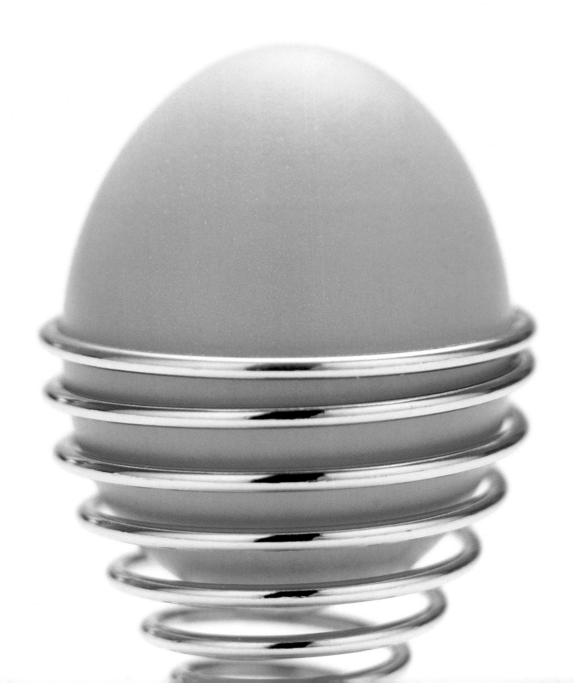

Banana Pecan

Muffins

Bananas make one of the best muffins, with a lovely moist texture and a natural sweetness that means you can cut down on the sugar. Thanks to pecans, oat bran, and whole-wheat flour, these are especially nutritious.

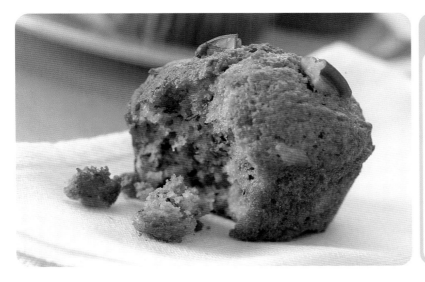

Nutritional guidance
Per muffin

206 calories
4 g protein
11 g fat (5 g saturated fat)
24 g carbohydrate
2 g fiber
152 mg sodium

✔✔   phosphorus, vitamin B12
✔   vitamin A

Makes 12 • Preparation time: 20 minutes • Cooking time: 20 minutes

1 cup all-purpose flour	Pinch of salt	1 teaspoon vanilla extract
1 teaspoon baking powder	⅓ cup soft light brown sugar	3 ripe bananas, mashed
1 teaspoon baking soda	½ cup pecans, chopped	1 stick sweet butter, melted
¾ cup whole-wheat flour	2 eggs	
¼ cup oat bran	4 tablespoons milk	

1   Preheat the oven to 375°F. Sift the all-purpose flour, baking powder, and baking soda into a bowl. Stir in the whole-wheat flour, oat bran, salt, sugar, and nuts and make a well in the center.

2   Whisk together the eggs, milk, and vanilla, then whisk in the mashed bananas and melted butter. Pour the wet ingredients into the well in the flour mixture and mix briefly until the ingredients are just combined (don't overmix or the muffins will be heavy).

3   Spoon the mixture into 12 greased muffin cups, or into paper baking cups, and bake for about 20 minutes, until the muffins are well risen and a skewer inserted in the center comes out clean.

4   Cool slightly in the pan, then turn out onto a wire rack to cool completely.

NOTE: These muffins can be frozen.

Raisin Bran
Muffins

If you mix all the dry ingredients together the night before, it does not take very long to make these muffins for breakfast in the morning.

Makes 12 • Preparation time: 15 minutes • Cooking time: 20 minutes

¾ cup all-purpose flour
2 teaspoons baking soda
Pinch of salt
¼ teaspoon ground cinnamon
¾ cup whole-wheat flour

¼ cup oat bran
⅓ cup dark brown sugar
¾ cup raisins
1 cup yogurt or buttermilk
½ stick sweet butter, melted

2 eggs
1 teaspoon vanilla extract
Grated zest of ½ lemon

1 Preheat the oven to 400°F. Sift the all-purpose flour, baking soda, salt, and cinnamon into a large bowl and stir in the whole-wheat flour, oat bran, sugar, and raisins.

2 Whisk together the yogurt or buttermilk, melted butter, eggs, vanilla, and lemon zest. Add this to the flour mixture and stir with a wooden spoon until just combined. Be careful not to overmix or the muffins will be heavy.

3 Spoon the mixture into 12 greased muffin cups, or into paper baking cups, and bake in the oven for about 20 minutes, until the muffins are well risen and golden brown.

4 Remove from the oven and allow to cool in the pan for a few minutes, then turn out onto a wire rack and allow to cool completely.

NOTE: These muffins can be frozen.

Nutritional guidance
Per serving

152 calories
4 g protein
5 g fat (2.5 g saturated fat)
26 g carbohydrate
2.5 g fiber
213 mg sodium

✔ phosphorus, iron

Buttermilk

Soda Bread

This must be the quickest ever bread to make. And if you're wondering whether it's worth making your own bread when it's so easy to buy, the answer is most definitely yes. Homemade bread tastes and smells better than the mass-produced version, and you can tailor it to suit your own nutritional needs and preferences – see below for suggestions.

If buttermilk is unavailable, substitute warm milk soured by the addition of about 1 tablespoon lemon juice and allowed to stand for 10 minutes.

Preparation time: 5 minutes • Cooking time: 40 minutes

3 cups whole-wheat flour	1 teaspoon salt	$1^1/_2$ to $1^3/_4$ cups buttermilk
1 cup all-purpose flour	1 teaspoon baking soda	

---

1 Preheat the oven to 400°F.

2 Put the flours, salt, and baking soda in a large bowl and stir together well. Stir in enough buttermilk to make a soft, slightly sticky dough. Turn out on to a floured surface and knead lightly – just for a minute or two, until smooth.

3 Shape into a round about 2 inches thick, place on a greased baking sheet, and cover with a deep cake pan (this is not essential but helps to produce a moist loaf). Bake for 35 minutes, then remove the cake pan or casserole and bake for about a further 5 minutes, until the bread is browned on top and sounds hollow when tapped underneath.

4 Leave on a wire rack to cool. This bread does not keep for more than a day or two but toasts well and can be frozen.

VARIATIONS:
- Replace $^1/_2$ to 1 cup of the flour with oat bran, oatmeal, rolled oats, wheat germ, or any combination of these.
- Sitr together flours, 2 tablespoons superfine sugar, $^1/_2$ cup mixed golden raisins and currants, and $^1/_4$ cup chopped mixed candied peel. Stir 2 tablespoons melted butter into the buttermilk and pour into the flour mixture. Combine well.
- Add 1 tablespoon caraway seeds or fennel seeds to the flour.

NOTE: This bread can be frozen.

> **Nutritional guidance**
> *Per serving*
>
> 1565 calories
> 67 g protein
> 11 g fat (2 g saturated fat)
> 320 g carbohydrate
> 35 g fiber
> 3284 mg sodium
>
> ---
>
> ✔✔ calcium
> ✔   iron, folate,
>   vitamin E

Bircher Muesli

with Fresh Berries

Bircher muesli was created by Dr. Bircher-Benner in the late 19th century to serve to patients at his clinic in Switzerland. Because the oats are soaked overnight, they are easily digested, and the addition of nuts, fresh and dried fruits, and honey make this a very nutritious dish. Muesli is also known as granola. Almost any fruits can be used instead of berries – peaches are delicious.

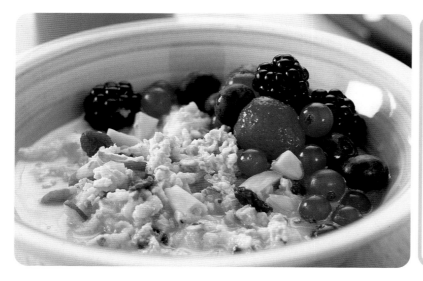

Nutritional guidance
Per serving

438 calories
13 g protein
13 g fat (2 g saturated fat)
72 g carbohydrate
7.5 g fiber
64 mg sodium

✔✔ phosphorus, calcium
✔ vitamin C, iron, vitamin B2, vitamin E

Serves 1 • Preparation time: 5 minutes, plus soaking overnight

4 tablespoons rolled oats
1 tablespoon golden raisins
6 tablespoons milk
1 small apple

2 teaspoons chopped almonds or hazelnuts
1 teaspoon honey

¼ to ½ cup berries – choose from raspberries, strawberries, blueberries, blackberries, or red currants
Yogurt, to serve (optional)

1 Put the oats and golden raisins in a bowl, add the milk, then cover and leave in the refrigerator overnight.

2 The next day, grate the apple and stir it into the oats with the nuts and honey.

3 Sprinkle the berries on top, add a spoonful or more of yogurt if desired, and eat immediately.

Sweet Cinnamon

Couscous

Couscous may seem an odd choice for breakfast. However, prepared this way it is like a cross between oatmeal and rice pudding and, in my view, nicer than either. It makes an excellent substantial snack or meal at any time of day when you don't feel like cooking. Serve topped with fresh fruit and Greek yogurt.

Serves 1 • Preparation time: 5 minutes, plus 10 minutes standing

1 cup couscous
5 dried apricots, chopped
1 tablespoon golden raisins

$^2/_3$ cup milk, plus extra to serve
Pinch of ground cinnamon

Raw brown sugar or maple syrup, to serve

1 Put the couscous, apricots, and golden raisins in a bowl. Put the milk and cinnamon in a small saucepan and bring to a boil, then pour it over the couscous. Cover the bowl with plastic wrap and allow to stand for 10 minutes.

2 Fluff up the couscous with a fork, pour over a little extra milk, then sprinkle over some brown sugar or drizzle over maple syrup.

Nutritional guidance
Per serving

362 calories
11.5 g protein
3 g fat (1.5 g saturated fat)
76 g carbohydrate
3.5 g fiber
106 mg sodium

✔✔   iron, calcium
✔   vitamin B1

Blueberry and Banana

Pancakes

These light, little pancakes have an intense fruit flavor, with bananas mixed into the batter and blueberries sprinkled on top during cooking. Have these for breakfast and they will perk you up for the rest of the day.

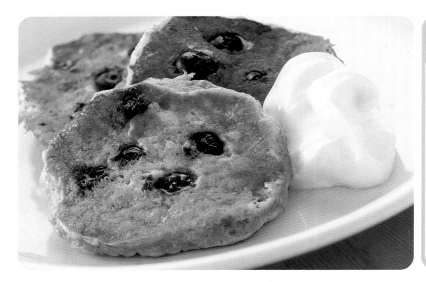

Nutritional guidance
For 3 pancakes

53 calories
2 g protein
1 g fat (0.3 g saturated fat)
10 g carbohydrate
0.5 g fiber
30 mg sodium

✔✔   vitamin B6
✔   calcium,
     phosphorus,
     vitamin B12

Makes about 18 • Preparation time: 10 minutes • Cooking time: 15 minutes

3 ripe bananas (overripe ones
   work best)
2 tablespoons sugar
2 teaspoons lemon juice
2 eggs, separated

1 cup self-rising flour, sifted
Pinch of ground cinnamon
Small pinch of salt
1 tablespoon peanut oil
1 cup blueberries

1   Mash the bananas with a fork in a large bowl. Use the fork to mix in the sugar, lemon juice, and egg yolks, followed by the flour and cinnamon.

2   In a separate bowl, whisk the egg whites and salt until stiff. Fold them into the banana mixture with a large metal spoon.

3   Heat about 1 tablespoon peanut oil in a large, heavy-based skillet over medium heat (you will need enough oil to coat the skillet in a very thin layer when it is hot). Drop in tablespoonfuls of the mixture to make pancakes and when they have been cooking for about a minute, sprinkle four to five blueberries on to each one, pushing them lightly into the batter. Cook for about 2 minutes longer, until browned underneath, then flip them over and cook the other side for a minute or so only, until lightly browned.

4   Transfer to a warm plate and cook the remaining pancakes.

French Toast

with Raspberries

This is a delicate, summery version of a breakfast favorite. If raspberries aren't available, try strawberries or blueberries instead – or even sliced banana.

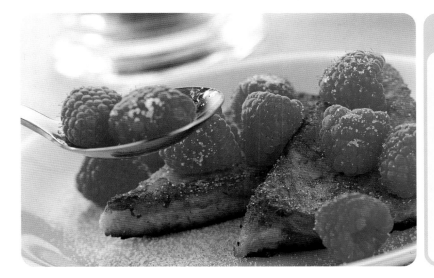

Nutritional guidance
Per serving

325 calories
13 g protein
10 g fat (5 g saturated fat)
50 g carbohydrate
3 g fiber
489 mg sodium

✔ calcium, vitamin B12, folate, vitamin C

Serves 2 • Preparation time: 10 minutes • Cooking time: 15 minutes

²/₃ cup raspberries
3 teaspoons sugar, plus extra for sprinkling
1 egg

¹/₂ cup milk
Generous pinch of ground cinnamon
Butter for frying

4 slices day-old white bread, or challah or brioche, crusts removed

1 Mix the raspberries with 1 teaspoon of the sugar and set aside.

2 Whisk together the egg, milk, cinnamon, and remaining sugar and pour into a shallow dish.

3 Cut the bread slices in half to make triangles and dip them into the egg mixture until saturated.

4 Heat a little butter in a skillet until gently sizzling. Fry the bread triangles in the butter until crisp and lightly colored on the outside.

5 Serve the toasted triangles hot, with the raspberries sprinkled on top.

Rhubarb, Ginger, and Orange *Compote*

Rhubarb and ginger make a fairly bracing start to the day, but at the same time this compote is light enough to tempt a delicate appetite. Make it the night before and serve chilled – it will keep in the refrigerator for 3 to 4 days.

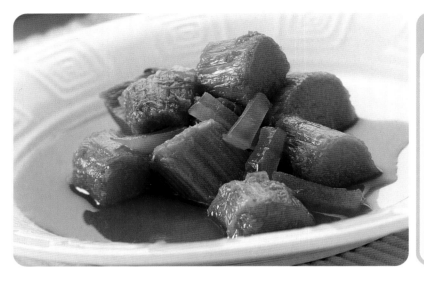

Nutritional guidance
Per serving

123 calories
1 g protein
0.1 g fat (0 g saturated fat)
32 g carbohydrate
2 g fiber
14 mg sodium

✔✔ vitamin C
✔   calcium

Serves 4 • Preparation time: 20 minutes • Cooking time: 45 to 60 minutes

1 pound rhubarb
¹/₃ cup soft brown sugar
Juice of 2 oranges

3 tablespoons fine sliced candied ginger in syrup, or to taste
Yogurt, or light cream, to serve

1 Preheat the oven to 300°F.

2 Trim the rhubarb and slice it into 1-inch pieces on the diagonal. Layer in a baking dish with the sugar, then pour over the orange juice and, if necessary, add a little water so that the liquid comes about three-quarters of the way up the rhubarb. Cover and bake for 45 to 60 minutes, until the rhubarb is tender but still holding its shape.

3 Remove from the oven, strain off the juice into a saucepan, and simmer until reduced and slightly syrupy.

4 Pour the juice over the rhubarb, stir in the candied ginger, and allow to cool.

5 Serve chilled, with yogurt or light cream.

NOTE: This compote can be frozen.

Vanilla Apple Compote

with Honeyed Greek Yogurt

This is a clever way of using up apples that have been sitting in the fruit bowl rather too long. The vanilla could be replaced with $1/2$ teaspoon ground cinnamon, or you could add a handful of golden raisins to the finished compote. It will keep well in the refrigerator for several days.

Serves 4 • Preparation time: 20 minutes • Cooking time: 30 minutes to $1^1/_4$ hours

2 pounds sweet, firm apples
1 teaspoon vanilla extract

2 tablespoons honey, or to taste
1 cup Greek yogurt

1 Peel, core, and chop the apples, discarding any bruised bits. Put them in a heavy-based saucepan with the vanilla and 2 tablespoons water.

2 Place over medium heat until they are hot, then turn the heat down as low as possible, cover with a tight-fitting lid, and cook until they are completely broken down. This can take anything from 30 minutes to $1^1/_4$ hours, depending on the type of apple and the heat level. Check regularly that they are not sticking to the base of the saucepan, stirring them and adding a little more water if necessary.

3 Once the apples are soft and pulpy, remove from the heat and beat them to a smooth purée with a wooden spoon.

4 Stir the honey into the yogurt and serve with the apple compote – it's good either hot or cold.

NOTE: This compote can be frozen.

Nutritional guidance
Per serving

186 calories
3 g protein
4 g fat (3 g saturated fat)
35 g carbohydrate
4 g fiber
92.5 mg sodium

✔ vitamin C, calcium, phosphorus

Juice Bar Treats

To make these juices, you will need to invest in a centrifugal juice extractor – a great piece of equipment. The juices it produces taste remarkably intense and potent, and you can almost feel them doing you good.

Below are just a few simple ideas for juices.

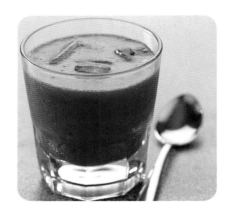

Celery, Carrot, and Beet

Serves 1

2 large carrots
1 beet, 2 to 3 inches in
    diameter

1 large or 2 small stalks
    celery

1 You don't really need to peel the vegetables, but by the time you have scrubbed them clean, you might as well just peel them. Cut the carrots, beet, and celery into pieces.

2 Push everything through the juicer.

3 Pour the juice onto crushed ice and serve.

Nutritional guidance
Per serving

136 calories
3.5 g protein
1 g fat (0.3 g saturated fat)
30 g carbohydrate
9 g fiber
154 mg sodium

✔✔   folate, vitamin A
✔   vitamin C, iron,
     vitamin E

Melon, Strawberry, and Apple

Serves 2

½ melon, such as Galia,
    Charentais, or Cantaloupe

1 apple
½ cup strawberries

1 Remove the peel and seeds from the melon and cut the flesh into large chunks.

2 Remove the stem from the apple and cut it into quarters. Hull the strawberries.

3 Push everything through the juicer, then pour the juice onto crushed ice and serve.

Nutritional guidance
Per serving

145 calories
3 g protein
0.5 g fat (0 g saturated fat)
34.5 g carbohydrate
4 g fiber
95 mg sodium

✔✔   vitamin C

Banana Berry Slush

You can use a blender for this one if you prefer, although the resulting juice will be full of seeds. The seeds are high in fiber, but if you prefer to omit them, strain the juice prior to drinking.

Serves 1

1 large ripe banana

About 1¼ cups mixed berries, including about ½ cup blackberries

1 Peel the banana and cut it into chunks.

2 Put everything in the blender and purée until smooth.

3 Pour the juice onto crushed ice, or, if you prefer strain to remove the seeds, then serve.

Nutritional guidance
Per serving

199 calories
5 g protein
1 g fat (0.2 g saturated fat)
45 g carbohydrate
8.5 g fiber
13 mg sodium

✔✔   vitamin C
✔   folate, vitamin E

Carrot, Apple, and Ginger

Serves 1 generously

2 carrots
2 sweet, firm apples

1 piece gingerroot, about ¼ inch thick

1 Scrub or peel the carrots and cut them into large pieces.

2 Remove the stems from the apples and cut them into wedges (there is no need to peel them or remove the cores).

3 Push the carrots and apples through the juicer, followed by the gingerroot.

4 Stir the juice thoroughly, then taste it and add more gingerroot if necessary.

5 Pour the juice onto crushed ice and serve.

Nutritional guidance
Per serving

199 calories
3 g protein
1 g fat (0.3 g saturated fat)
47 g carbohydrate
10 g fiber
78 mg sodium

✔✔   vitamin A
✔   vitamin C, vitamin E

Breakfast in a Glass

This is something you can prepare quickly when you don't feel like eating anything substantial.

Serves 1 • Preparation time: 5 minutes

1 teaspoon sunflower seeds
1 teaspoon sesame seeds
1 ripe banana, sliced

5 tablespoons yogurt
5 tablespoons milk
2 teaspoons honey

1 Grind the sunflower and sesame seeds to a powder – a coffee grinder is good for this, or a mini food processor.

2 Put the ground seeds in a blender with all the remaining ingredients and blend until smooth.

3 Pour into a glass and drink immediately.

VARIATION: If you are really in a hurry, plain banana milk is even quicker to make: just slice one ripe banana into a blender, add enough milk to cover the blades generously, and blend until frothy. Sprinkle a little freshly grated nutmeg on top.

Nutritional guidance
Per serving

340 calories
16 g protein
8 g fat (2 g saturated fat)
55 g carbohydrate
2 g fiber
211 mg sodium

✔✔ calcium
✔ vitamin C, vitamin E

Oatmeal with Milk and Honey

A variation on the traditional Scottish porridge, this is popular with those who usually find oatmeal too austere. You could also add a handful of golden raisins or a sliced banana.

Serves 1 • Preparation time: 5 minutes
• Cooking time: 5 minutes

$1/2$ cup oatmeal
$1 1/4$ cups reduced-fat milk

Pinch of salt
2 teaspoons honey

1 Put the oatmeal in a small saucepan, add the milk and salt, and bring slowly to a boil. Simmer for 1 to 2 minutes, stirring occasionally, then pour into a bowl.

2 Drizzle the honey on top and eat immediately, with extra milk if you like.

Nutritional guidance
Per serving

350 calories
15 g protein
9 g fat (4 g saturated fat)
57 g carbohydrate
3 g fiber
167 mg sodium

✔✔ calcium, phosphorus, vitamin B2
✔ iron, vitamin B1, vitamin B6

Salsa Verde

Omelet

This takes only a couple of minutes to prepare and contains cottage cheese for extra calcium. Many women enjoy spicy foods at some stage of their pregnancy, but if you don't feel up to it yet, substitute 2 to 3 tablespoons chopped herbs for the salsa verde.

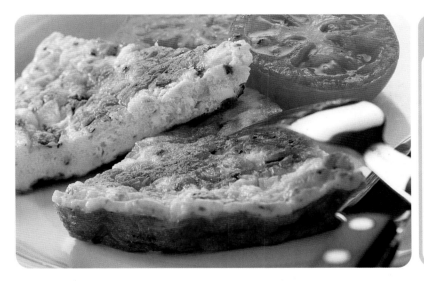

Nutritional guidance
Per serving

164 calories
13 g protein
12 g fat (3 g saturated fat)
2 g carbohydrate
0.1 g fiber
398 mg sodium

✔✔   calcium,
       phosphorus,
       vitamin B12
✔   iron,
       vitamin A

Serves 4 • Preparation time: 2 minutes • Cooking time: 15 minutes

¹/₂ cup cottage cheese
2 tablespoons Mexican-style salsa verde, or to taste

5 eggs
1 tablespoon olive oil

Salt and freshly ground black pepper

1   Mix the cottage cheese and salsa together with a fork, then whisk in the eggs. Season with a little salt and pepper.

2   Heat the olive oil in an 8-inch skillet over medium heat. Pour in the egg mixture, reduce the heat a little, and cook for about 10 minutes, until browned underneath and mostly set but still a little liquid on top.

3   Place under a hot broiler until completely set and lightly browned. Serve hot, warm, or cold, with broiled tomatoes.

Salads and Soups

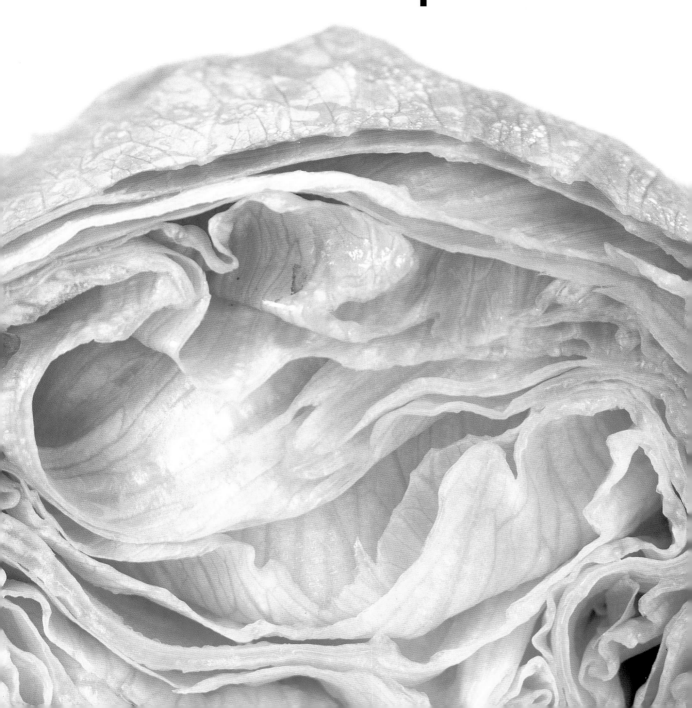

Lentil, Roasted Bell Pepper, and Broccoli

Salad

French green lentils have a good nutty flavor and keep their shape well, making them ideal to use in salads. Lentils are rich in iron, and the vitamin C in the bell peppers, lemon, and broccoli helps ensure that your body can absorb it.

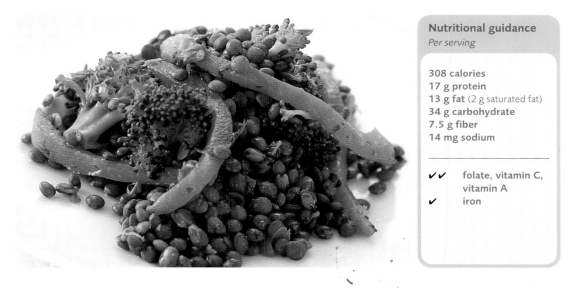

Nutritional guidance
Per serving

308 calories
17 g protein
13 g fat (2 g saturated fat)
34 g carbohydrate
7.5 g fiber
14 mg sodium

✔✔   folate, vitamin C, vitamin A
✔   iron

Serves 4 • Preparation time: 20 minutes • Cooking time: 25 minutes

2 red bell peppers
³/₄ cup small broccoli florets
1¹/₃ cup French green lentils
1 bay leaf

4 tablespoons olive oil
2 tablespoons lemon juice
Pinch of cayenne pepper
1 clove garlic, minced
2 tablespoons chopped mint

1 tablespoon chopped flat-leaf parsley
Salt and freshly ground black pepper

1   Put the red bell peppers under a hot broiler and broil until blackened and blistered all over, turning as necessary. Leave until cool enough to handle, then peel off the skin and discard the seeds. Cut the bell peppers into thin strips, reserving any juices, and set aside.

2   Steam or boil the broccoli florets until tender then drain well and set aside.

3   Put the lentils in a saucepan with the bay leaf and cover generously with water. Bring to a boil and simmer for 20 to 25 minutes, until just tender, then drain well and transfer to a wide shallow dish.

4   Whisk together the oil, lemon juice, cayenne pepper, garlic, and some salt and pepper. Pour this dressing over the hot lentils and mix well.

5   Stir in the mint and parsley, followed by the red bell peppers and their juice, and the broccoli. Serve at room temperature, but not chilled.

Trout and Flageolet Bean Salad
with Walnut Vinaigrette

This pretty, pale pink and green salad makes a good light meal or appetizer. Serve with plenty of crusty bread to mop up the juices.

Serves 2 • Preparation time: 20 minutes • Cooking time: 15 to 20 minutes

1 trout, weighing about 10 ounces
2 lemon slices
2 sprigs parsley
14-ounce can flageolet beans
2 small to medium tomatoes, skinned, seeded, and cut into ¼-inch dice

1 tablespoon chopped chives or parsley
¼ cup walnuts, broken up and roasted lightly in a dry skillet
Salt and freshly ground black pepper

For the vinaigrette:
1 tablespoon walnut oil
1 tablespoon olive oil
1 tablespoon white wine vinegar
½ small clove garlic, minced

1 Preheat the oven to 375°F.

2 Put the trout on a large piece of oiled foil, insert the lemon slices and parsley sprigs in the cavity, and season inside and out with salt and pepper. Wrap loosely in the foil and bake for 15 to 20 minutes (to check if the trout is done, insert a knife near the backbone; the flesh should flake but still be moist). Allow to cool. Remove the skin and bones, separate the flesh into chunks, and season well with salt and pepper.

3 Drain the beans, rinse well, and pat dry on paper towels. Put them in a shallow dish with the diced tomatoes.

4 **To prepare the vinaigrette:** Whisk together all the ingredients for the vinaigrette, season well with salt and pepper, and toss about three-quarters of it with the beans.

5 Stir in most of the chives and parsley and most of the trout, saving a few chunks of trout to garnish. Arrange these on top of the salad, then sprinkle over the walnuts and the remaining herbs, drizzle over the remaining dressing, and serve.

NOTE: If canned beans are not available, use 1 cup frozen small lima beans, cooked according to the package directions, and allowed to cool.

Nutritional guidance
Per serving

462 calories
38 g protein
24 g fat (3 g saturated fat)
24 g carbohydrate
9 g fiber
540 mg sodium

✔✔ vitamin D
✔ vitamin C,
vitamin A,
vitamin E,
calcium, iron

Fennel, Orange, and Black Olive

Salad

A French friend once told me that her mother always made a point of providing something raw to start a meal, even if it was only some grated carrot or a few crudités. It is a good habit to get into, and this refreshing salad fits the bill perfectly. It's quick to prepare, full of goodness, and stimulates the appetite.

Serves 2 • Preparation time: 10 minutes

1 large fennel bulb	1 tablespoon olive oil	Salt and freshly ground black pepper
2 oranges	Handful black olives, used whole	

1   Trim the fennel bulb, removing the outer layers and long stalks. Reserve any feathery fronds, then cut the bulb in half and cut out the core. Thinly slice the fennel halves crosswise and place in a shallow serving dish.

2   Cut off all the peel and pith from the oranges. Hold one orange over the fennel and cut down one side of a segment to separate it from the membrane, then cut down the other side, allowing the segment to fall onto the fennel.

3   Remove the remaining segments in the same way, turning back the flaps of membrane like the pages of a book. Once you have removed all the segments, squeeze the membrane gently so some of the juice runs over the fennel – you don't need much, just enough to moisten it. Repeat with the second orange.

4   Drizzle the olive oil over the fennel and orange, and season with salt and pepper. Mix together well, then sprinkle the olives on top and any fronds reserved from the fennel. Serve immediately.

Nutritional guidance
Per serving

150 calories
3 g protein
8 g fat (1 g saturated fat)
16 g carbohydrate
7 g fiber
531 mg sodium

✔✔   vitamin C
✔   calcium, folate

Potato and Arugula Salad

with Pesto Dressing and Roasted Corn

You don't have to include the roasted corn, but it is a remarkably good way of preparing it and makes a good contrast to the potatoes and arugula. This salad makes a satisfying meal in itself, served with some bread, or it can be served as an accompaniment to broiled meat.

Serves 2 • Preparation time: 15 minutes, plus 20 minutes soaking • Cooking time: 50 minutes

1 corn on the cob
Olive oil

1¹⁄₂ pounds new potatoes, peeled
2 tablespoons good-quality pesto
Lemon juice

Generous handful arugula leaves

1 Preheat the oven to 375°F.

2 Soak the corn on the cob in cold water for 20 minutes, then drain and pat dry on paper towels. Brush with olive oil, place in a roasting dish, and roast for about 50 minutes, until golden and slightly wrinkled. Leave until cool enough to handle, then stand the corn cob upright on a board and slice off the kernels. Set aside.

3 Cook the potatoes in boiling salted water until tender, then drain well. Set aside.

4 Thin down the pesto to coating consistency with olive oil and lemon juice to taste, then toss with the hot potatoes. Mix in the corn and then carefully toss in the arugula leaves so that they become coated with the dressing and just wilt in the heat. Serve immediately.

> **Nutritional guidance**
> *Per serving*
>
> 445 calories
> 13.5 g protein
> 16 g fat (4 g saturated fat)
> 66 g carbohydrate
> 5 g fiber
> 164 mg sodium
>
> ✔✔   vitamin C
> ✔   folate, vitamin A

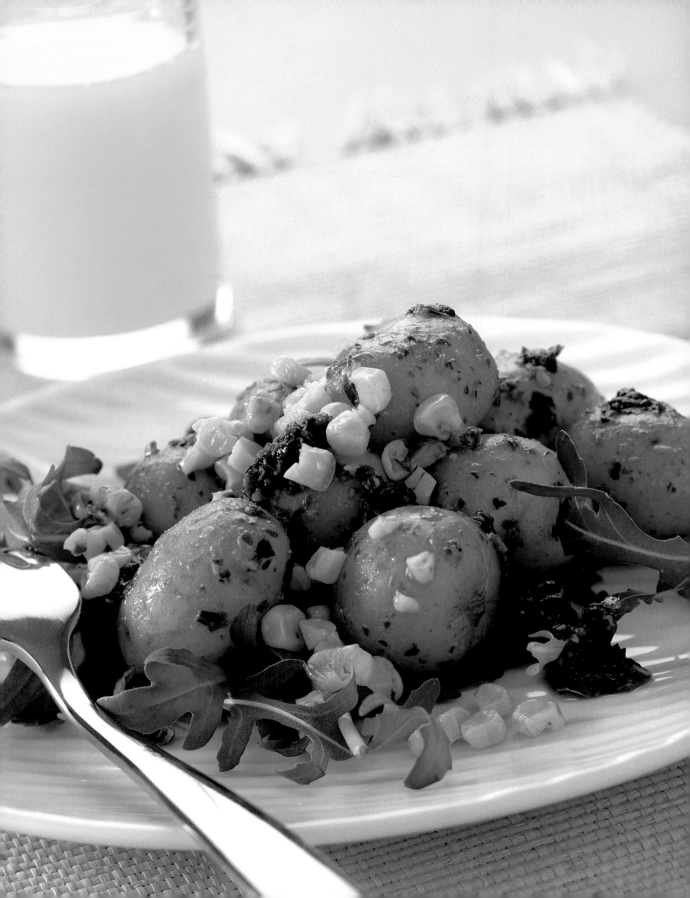

Watercress, Avocado, and Pink Grapefruit *Salad*

This pretty salad makes a good appetizer. Avocados are high in fat, albeit mainly monounsaturated, and are a real package of goodness, containing vitamins A, B6, C, and E, plus potassium and protein, so it's worth including avocados in your diet if possible.

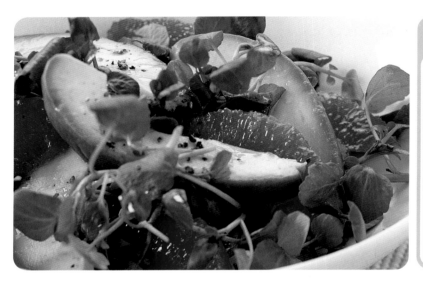

Nutritional guidance
Per serving

335 calories
4 g protein
30 g fat (6 g saturated fat)
12 g carbohydrate
6 g fiber
29 mg sodium

✔✔ vitamin C,
     vitamin E
✔   vitamin A,
     calcium,
     phosphorus

Serves 2 • Preparation time: 15 minutes

1 large pink grapefruit	1 teaspoon sherry vinegar	1 large ripe avocado
1 tablespoon olive oil	3 cups watercress, large stalks	Salt and freshly ground black
1 tablespoon peanut oil	removed	pepper

1 Cut off all the peel and pith from the grapefruit. Cut down one side of a grapefruit segment to separate it from the membrane, then cut down the other side and remove the segment. Remove the remaining segments in the same way, turning back the flaps of membrane like the pages of a book.

2 Once you have removed all the segments, squeeze out the membrane into a small bowl to collect the juice (there should be about 2 tablespoonfuls). Add the olive oil, peanut oil, sherry vinegar, and some salt and pepper, and whisk until emulsified. Taste, and add a little more oil, vinegar, or seasoning if necessary. Set aside.

3 Put the watercress in a bowl and toss with half the dressing, then divide it between two serving plates.

4 Cut the avocado in half, pit, and peel, then cut each half lengthwise into thin slices. Fan them out on top of the watercress, then arrange the grapefruit segments over them, so you can see both pink and green.

5 Season lightly with salt and pepper, drizzle over the remaining dressing, and serve immediately.

High-vitality

Green Salad

Most of the time I was pregnant, I found it hard to eat anything green, but this salad was an exception. Fennel and mint give it a fresh flavor, while butter lettuce and pine nuts lend an unexpected sweetness. There's no need to drown it in a complicated salad dressing – all you need is a little olive oil and the best-quality red wine vinegar to enhance the flavors.

Serves 2 to 4 • Preparation time: 10 minutes

$^1/_2$ small fennel bulb
2-inch piece cucumber
1 butter lettuce
3 cups mixed salad leaves, such as arugula, spinach, lettuce

$^1/_2$ avocado, peeled and cubed (optional)
1 tablespoon chopped mint
1 tablespoon chopped flat-leaf parsley
1 teaspoon chopped chives
2 to 3 tablespoons olive oil

1 teaspoon good-quality red wine vinegar
$1^1/_2$ tablespoons pine nuts, lightly roasted
Salt and freshly ground black pepper

1   Trim the fennel, slice it thin, and place in a salad bowl.

2   Slice the cucumber very thin and add to the bowl.

3   Roughly tear the large outer leaves of the butter lettuce, and then slice the inner core into chunks. Add to the salad bowl with the mixed salad leaves.

4   Add the avocado, if using; sprinkle the mint, parsley, and chives on top, and season to taste with salt and pepper

5   Toss the salad with just enough olive oil to coat each leaf lightly – they should just be lubricated, not wet. Sprinkle over the vinegar and toss well again.

6   Garnish with the roasted pine nuts and serve immediately.

Nutritional guidance
Per serving

153 calories
3 g protein
14.5 g fat (2 g saturated fat)
3 g carbohydrate
3 g fiber
27 mg sodium

✔   folate, phosphorus, vitamin C

Couscous Salad

with Chargrilled Chicken

Plenty of lemon juice, summer herbs, and a touch of harissa ensure that the flavors of this salad are clean and fresh. Harissa is a red-hot paste from North Africa, available in jars, from specialty stores or markets.

Serves 4 • Preparation time: 30 minutes, plus 1 hour marinating • Cooking time: about 10 minutes

4 chicken breasts
1 clove garlic, minced
Olive oil
Juice of $\frac{1}{2}$ lemon
Salt and freshly ground black pepper

For the couscous salad:
$1\frac{1}{4}$ cups couscous
1 teaspoon harissa paste
1 cup water, at boiling point
2 tablespoons olive oil
4 tablespoons lemon juice
5 tablespoons fine chopped mint

2 tablespoons fine chopped flat-leaf parsley
2 tablespoons fine chopped cilantro
2- to 3-inch piece cucumber
1 cup small, firm cherry tomatoes, cut in half

1 Put the chicken breasts in a shallow dish and sprinkle over the garlic. Drizzle with olive oil, then pour over the lemon juice and season with black pepper. Cover with plastic wrap and leave to marinate for about an hour.

2 Meanwhile, make the salad. Put the couscous into a large bowl. Stir the harissa into the boiling water and pour the water over the couscous. Cover the bowl with a dishtowel and allow to stand for 15 to 20 minutes for the couscous to soften. Fluff the couscous up with a fork, breaking up any lumps with your fingers, then mix in the olive oil, lemon juice, and mint, parsley, and cilantro.

3 Peel the cucumber, cut it lengthwise into quarters, and scrape out the seeds. Slice the cucumber into thin strips, and stir it into the salad together with the tomatoes. Season to taste with salt and pepper, adding more lemon juice if necessary.

4 Heat a ridged grill pan over medium-high heat, add the chicken, skin-side down, and cook until it is nicely scored with lines from the grill. Turn the chicken over, reduce the heat a little, and continue to grill until it is cooked through. Remove from the grill pan and allow to rest for about 10 minutes, then slice on the diagonal.

5 Divide the couscous between four serving plates, top with the chicken, and serve.

Nutritional guidance
Per serving

311 calories
28 g protein
9 g fat (1 g saturated fat)
31 g carbohydrate
1 g fiber
86 mg sodium

✔✔ phosphorus,
✔   vitamin C, iron

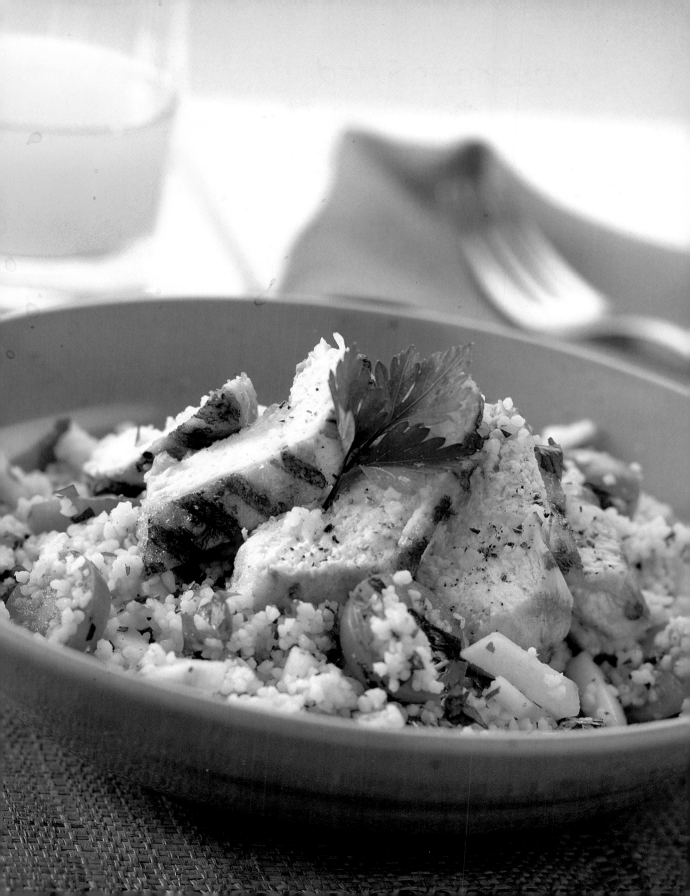

Potato, Avocado, and Bacon Salad
with Mustard Dressing

This warm salad makes a quick and satisfying supper dish.

Serves 2 • Preparation time: 20 minutes • Cooking time: about 25 minutes

1 pound small boiling potatoes
3 tablespoons olive oil
3 slices bacon, chopped

1 large tomato, skinned, seeded, and diced
1½ tablespoons red wine vinegar
1½ tablespoons Dijon mustard

1 ripe avocado, peeled, pitted, and diced
1 tablespoon chopped cilantro
Salt and freshly ground black pepper

1 Cook the potatoes in boiling salted water until tender, then drain. Leave until cool enough to handle, then peel, cut into chunks, and place in a salad bowl. Season with salt and pepper.

2 Heat 1 tablespoon of the olive oil in a skillet, add the bacon, and fry until crisp. Add the tomato, vinegar, and the remaining olive oil, and cook, stirring, for 1 minute. Stir in the mustard and simmer for 1 minute.

3 Pour this mixture over the hot potatoes and mix well, then carefully stir in the diced avocado. Sprinkle with the cilantro and serve immediately.

Nutritional guidance
Per serving

524 calories
14 g protein
35 g fat (7 g saturated fat)
41 g carbohydrate
5.5 g fiber
838 mg sodium

✔✔ vitamin C
✔ folate, vitamin A, vitamin E

Potato and Parsley

Soup

Parsley deserves to be more than just a garnish on the side of your plate. It is a useful source of iron and vitamin C, and this easy soup is a good way to enjoy its delicate flavor. It is a good soup to make after finishing a roast chicken; make a simple broth with the carcass (see page 96), and ladle it straight into the saucepan with the potatoes and parsley.

Serves 4 • Preparation time: 20 minutes • Cooking time: 45 minutes

$^1/_4$ stick butter or, if available, chicken or bacon fat
1 large onion, chopped
1 small leek, chopped
1 large clove garlic, chopped

1 pound potatoes, peeled and cut into 1-inch dice
Bunch of parsley, about 2 ounces, including stalks
4 cups good-quality chicken broth

Salt and freshly ground black pepper

1   Melt the butter in a large saucepan; add the onion, leek, and garlic; and cook gently for about 5 minutes, until softened.

2   Add the potatoes, stir to coat them in the butter, then cover and sweat for about 10 minutes.

3   Remove the stalks from the parsley, discarding any damaged bits, tear them roughly, and add to the saucepan.

4   Pour in the broth, then cover and cook for about 30 minutes, until the potatoes are very tender.

5   Stir in all of the parsley leaves except for about 2 tablespoonfuls, and cook for a few minutes longer.

6   Purée the soup in a blender, then return to the saucepan. Season well with salt and pepper, and reheat gently. Chop the remaining parsley leaves fine, and stir into the soup.

Nutritional guidance
Per serving

165 calories
4 g protein
6 g fat (3.5 g saturated fat)
26 g carbohydrate
4 g fiber
61 mg sodium

✔✔   vitamin C
✔   folate, vitamin A

Gingered *Chicken Noodle Soup*

This invigorating soup has a warm glow from the gingerroot. If you don't want anything too spicy, just omit the chile.

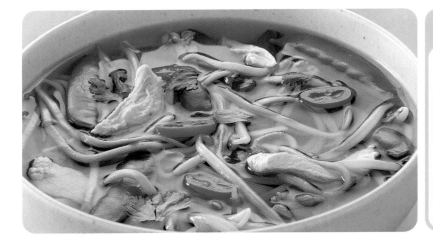

Nutritional guidance
Per serving

258 calories
25 g protein
4 g fat (1 g saturated fat)
32 g carbohydrate
2 g fiber
262 mg sodium

✔✔ phosphorus
✔   vitamin C, iron, zinc, vitamin B1, vitamin B12

Serves 2 • Preparation time: 15 minutes • Cooking time: 20 minutes

For the broth:
2-inch piece gingerroot, peeled
1 large clove garlic, peeled
2 stalks lemongrass
2$\frac{1}{2}$ pints good-quality chicken or vegetable broth
3 ounces egg noodles
$\frac{1}{2}$ cup sugar snap peas

1 chicken breast, skinned and shredded thin
Large handful bean sprouts
1 teaspoon fine chopped gingerroot
1 fresh red chile, seeded and cut into thin rings
1$\frac{1}{2}$ teaspoons Thai fish sauce (*nam pla*)

1$\frac{1}{2}$ teaspoons soy sauce
Pinch of sugar
Squeeze of lemon juice
1 heaping tablespoon cilantro leaves
1 heaping tablespoon mint leaves

1 **To prepare the broth:** Crush both the gingerroot and the garlic with the flat of a large knife, so they are pounded but left whole. Trim the lemongrass stalks, remove the hard outer layers, then crush the lemongrass with the flat part of the knife in the same way. Put these aromatics into a saucepan with the broth and bring to a boil. Simmer for 15 minutes, then strain into a clean saucepan, discarding the aromatics. Set aside.

2 Cook the noodles in a large saucepan of boiling water according to the instructions on the package, then drain and rinse with cold water. Set aside.

3 Bring the strained broth to a boil, and add the sugar snap peas. Bring back to a simmer and add the chicken. Cover and simmer gently for 1 to 2 minutes. Add the noodles, bean sprouts, gingerroot, and chile; mix well; and simmer for 1 minute. Stir in the fish sauce, soy sauce, sugar, and lemon juice, then taste and adjust the seasoning if necessary.

4 Tear over half the cilantro and mint leaves, and transfer the soup to two large, deep bowls.

5 Tear over the remaining cilantro and mint leaves, and serve immediately.

White Onion

Soup

This is a good soup to make when you have little food in the house. It doesn't take much more than a few onions, milk, and stale bread for crumbs, and proves that even a frugal selection of ingredients can produce something delicious.

Serves 4 • Preparation time: 15 minutes • Cooking time: $1^1/_2$ hours

3 tablespoons butter
$1^1/_2$ pounds white onions, sliced thin
$1/_2$ cup fresh white bread crumbs

$2^1/_2$ cups chicken or vegetable broth
$2^1/_2$ cups milk
Freshly grated nutmeg (optional)

Salt and freshly ground black pepper

1 Heat the butter in a large heavy-based pan, add the onions, then cover the saucepan and cook gently, stirring occasionally, for 40 to 60 minutes, until the onions are completely soft but not colored.

2 Add all the remaining ingredients and simmer gently for 45 minutes.

3 Purée in a blender, then return to the saucepan and reheat gently. Taste and adjust the seasoning, if necessary adding a little grated nutmeg if desired. Serve. This soup is good with grated cheese sprinkled on top.

NOTE: This soup can be frozen.

Nutritional guidance
Per serving

216 calories
7 g protein
11 g fat (7 g saturated fat)
24 g carbohydrate
2.5 g fiber
193 mg sodium

✔ calcium,
    vitamin A

Provençal Vegetable Soup

with Pistou

Pistou is the Provençal version of pesto, a basil paste that is stirred into this spring vegetable soup just before serving. You can use whatever vegetables are available to make this soup, and, if you have no fresh basil at hand, substitute a good-quality storebought pesto for the homemade pistou. It's worth making a large quantity of this soup because it will keep in the refrigerator for several days. Any leftover pistou can be tossed with pasta, stirred into mashed potatoes, or added to sandwiches.

Serves 6 • Preparation time: 30 minutes • Cooking time: 1¹/₂ hours

2 tablespoons olive oil
2 large onions, diced
2 carrots, diced
2 celery stalks, chopped
1 small turnip, diced (optional)
3 small zucchini, diced
2 cloves garlic, minced
2 small potatoes (about 9 ounces), diced

1 cup green beans, cut into 1-inch lengths
14-ounce can diced tomatoes
2 to 3 large sage leaves
2¹/₂ pints water
14-ounce can navy or cannellini beans, drained and rinsed
¹/₄ cup rice, small macaroni, or vermicelli

Salt and freshly ground black pepper

For the pistou:
2 large cloves garlic, chopped
¹/₂ teaspoon coarse salt
1 cup basil leaves
About 6 tablespoons olive oil
¹/₄ cup freshly grated Parmesan, plus extra to serve

1 Heat the oil in a large saucepan, add the onions, and cook gently for about 5 minutes, until softened but not colored. Add the carrots and celery, and cook until softened; then stir in the turnip, if using, plus the zucchini, garlic, potatoes, and green beans. Cook for about 5 minutes, stirring occasionally.

2 Add the canned tomatoes, sage, water, and some salt. Bring to a boil and simmer for about 1 hour, until the vegetables are tender and the liquid is slightly reduced.

3 Add the beans and the rice or pasta, and simmer for about 15 minutes, until the rice or pasta is tender. Add a little more water if the soup has become too thick, then season with salt and pepper to taste.

4 To prepare the pistou: Blend the garlic and salt together in a food processor, then add the basil and 1 tablespoon of the oil and blend again to make a paste. Add the cheese, then gradually pour in the oil, with the motor running, until the mixture has a fairly loose consistency.

5 Pour the soup into bowls, and spoon over pistou onto each one. Serve with extra grated Parmesan cheese and some crusty bread, if desired.

Nutritional guidance
Per serving

197 calories
8 g protein
5 g fat (1 g saturated fat)
33 g carbohydrate
6.5 g fiber
201 mg sodium

✔✔ vitamin A
✔ folate, vitamin C

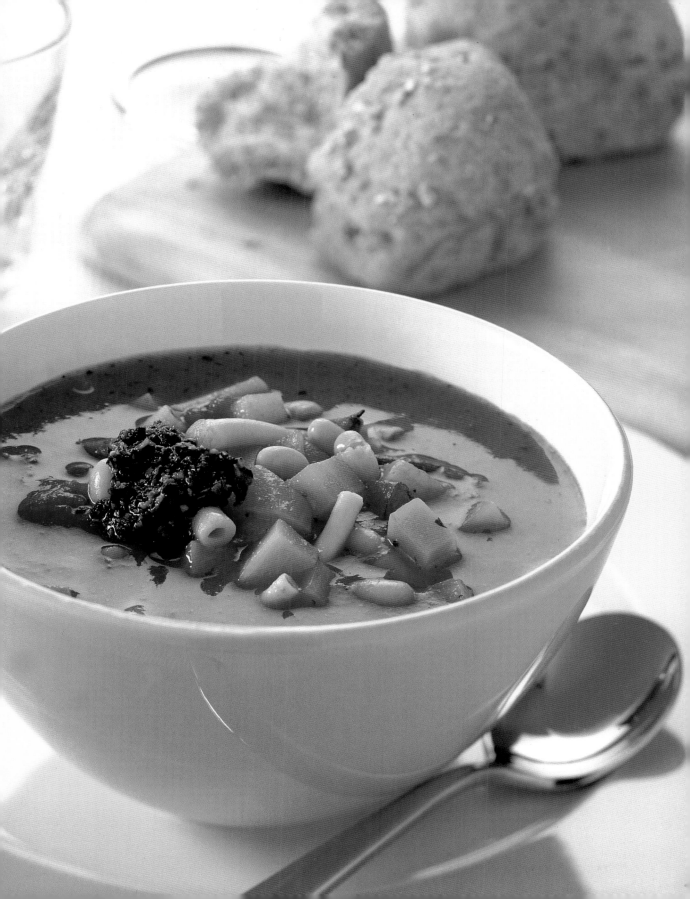

Watercress *Soup*

This makes a generous amount, but the soup can be stored in the refrigerator for 2 to 3 days and also freezes well, so is worth preparing in quantity. If you don't feel like eating anything rich, simply omit the cream; it is still a very soothing soup without it, spiked with the peppery flavor of watercress.

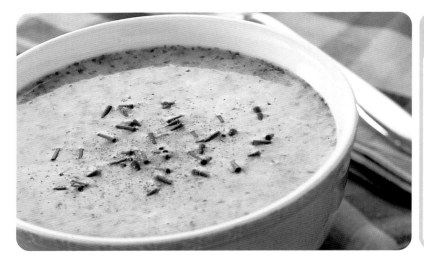

Nutritional guidance
Per serving

129 calories
5 g protein
4 g fat (2.5 g saturated fat)
20 g carbohydrate
1.5 g fiber
75 mg sodium

✔   calcium,
       phosphorus,
       vitamin A,
       vitamin B1

Serves 8 • Preparation time: 20 minutes • Cooking time: 45 minutes

¹/₄ stick butter
1 onion, chopped
1¹/₂ pounds potatoes, peeled and cut into ³/₄-inch dice
3 cups watercress

4 cups good-quality chicken or vegetable broth
2¹/₂ cups milk
²/₃ cup light cream (optional)
Freshly grated nutmeg

Salt and freshly ground black pepper
Chopped fresh chives, to garnish (optional)

1 Melt the butter in a large saucepan, add the onion, and sweat for about 5 minutes, until softened but not colored. Add the potatoes, cover, and cook gently for 8 to 10 minutes.

2 Meanwhile, remove and discard any large, tough stalks from the watercress, and set aside about a third of the leafy sprigs. Stir the remaining two-thirds of the watercress into the saucepan, and pour in the broth and milk. Bring to a boil and simmer for about 30 minutes, until the potatoes are tender.

3 Purée in a blender, adding the reserved watercress to the blender.

4 Return to the saucepan, add the cream, if using, and season to taste with nutmeg, salt, and pepper. If you are omitting the cream, you may need to thin the soup down with a little water, milk, or broth.

5 Reheat gently but do not allow the soup to boil. Serve garnished with chopped chives, if desired. The soup can also be served chilled.

NOTE: This soup can be frozen, either before or after adding the cream.

Spinach and Lentil Soup

with Preserved Lemons

Preserved lemons, available from some large supermarkets, specialty food stores, or Middle Eastern markets, give this nourishing soup a sharp, fresh flavor. Serve steaming hot, with pita or other Middle Eastern bread.

Serves 4 • Preparation time: 15 minutes • Cooking time: 40 minutes

2 tablespoons olive oil
1 large onion, sliced
2 cloves garlic, chopped fine
$1/2$ teaspoon ground coriander
$1/2$ teaspoon ground cumin

$1^1/_3$ cups brown or green lentils
$2^1/_2$ pints vegetable broth or water
1 pound young spinach

2 tablespoons chopped preserved lemons (use only the peel)
Pinch of cayenne pepper
Salt and freshly ground black pepper

1 Heat the olive oil in a large saucepan, add the onion and garlic, and fry until just beginning to brown.

2 Stir in the ground coriander and cumin, and cook for 1 minute; then stir in the lentils, followed by the broth or water. Bring to a boil and simmer for about 30 minutes, until the lentils are tender.

3 Wash the spinach and remove any large stalks. Drain in a colander, then add to the soup, pushing it down into the lentils. Cover the saucepan and cook for 2 to 3 minutes, until the spinach has wilted but is still bright green.

4 Stir in the chopped preserved lemons, season to taste with cayenne pepper, salt, and black pepper, then cook for a further minute before serving.

Nutritional guidance
Per serving

268 calories
18 g protein
8 g fat (1 g saturated fat)
34 g carbohydrate
8 g fiber
166 mg sodium

✔✔ folate, vitamin A
✔ calcium, iron, vitamin C

Carrot Soup
with Celery and Walnut Scones

Rice works well as a thickener in soups, giving this one a soothing texture. The scones make a delicious accompaniment. Any left over can be served as a snack with butter, cream cheese, or cottage cheese.

Serves 4 • Preparation time: 40 minutes • Cooking time: 45 to 60 minutes

1 tablespoon butter
1 small onion, chopped
1¼ pounds carrots, preferably young ones, sliced
2 tablespoons Italian short-grain rice, such as arborio
4 cups chicken or vegetable broth
Salt and freshly ground black pepper

For the celery and walnut scones:
1 cup all-purpose flour
1 cup whole-wheat flour
2 teaspoons baking powder
Pinch of cayenne pepper
Generous pinch of salt
3 tablespoons butter, diced
2 celery stalks, diced very fine
2 tablespoons chopped walnuts

1 cup grated Cheddar cheese
1 tablespoon chopped parsley
About ⅔ cup milk

1 Heat the butter in a large saucepan, add the onion, and sweat for about 5 minutes, until softened. Add the carrots and sweat for 10 to 15 minutes, then stir in the rice. Pour in the broth, bring to a boil, and simmer for 30 to 40 minutes, until the carrots are very soft.

2 Purée in a blender until smooth, then return to the saucepan, season to taste with salt and pepper, and reheat. If the soup is too thick, add a little broth or water.

3 To prepare the scones: Preheat the oven to 400°F.

4 Sift the flours, baking powder, cayenne pepper, and salt into a bowl, and rub in the butter with your fingertips until the mixture resembles fine crumbs. Stir in the celery, walnuts, cheese, and parsley, then add enough milk to make a soft but not sticky dough (you may not need all the milk).

5 Pat into a round at least 1 inch thick, and place on a greased baking sheet. Mark it into 6 or 8 wedges with a knife, then bake for about 25 minutes, until the scone round is risen and golden. Leave until just warm and serve with the soup.

NOTE: Both soup and scones can be frozen.

Nutritional guidance
Per serving

525 calories
16 g protein
27 g fat (14 g saturated fat)
57 g carbohydrate
7 g fiber
576 mg sodium

✔✔ vitamin A, phosphorus
✔ calcium

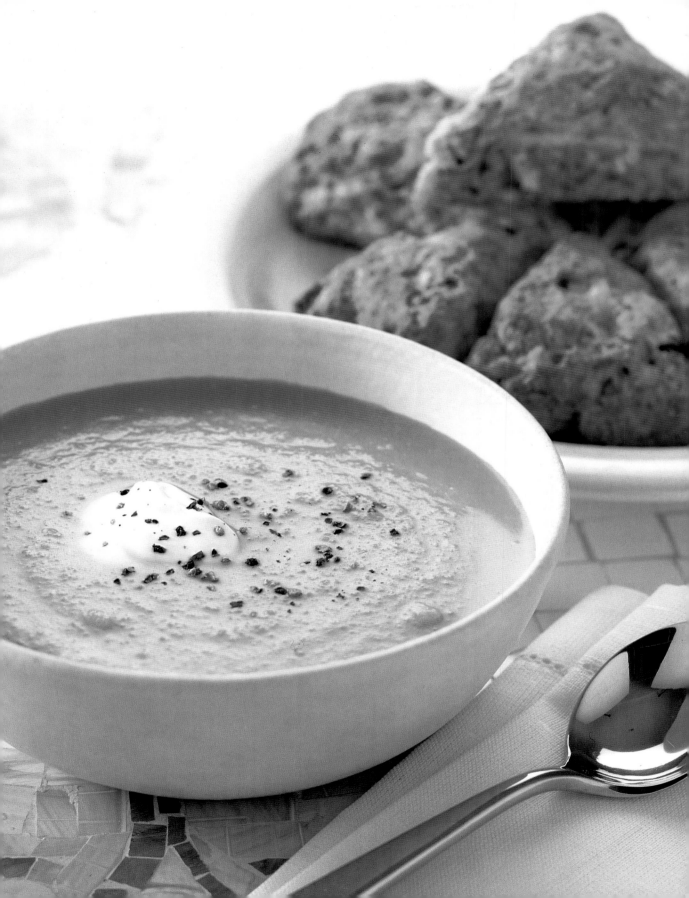

White Bean and Roasted Squash *Soup*

This hearty, richly flavored soup is so thick it is almost like a stew. If you prefer it thinner, just add a little more broth or water at the end.

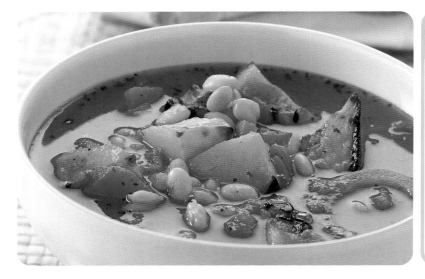

Nutritional guidance
Per serving

232 calories
10 g protein
6 g fat (1 g saturated fat)
36 g carbohydrate
9.5 g fiber
53 mg sodium

✔✔   vitamin A,
       vitamin E,
       vitamin B6
✔   calcium, folate,
       vitamin C, iron

Serves 6 • Preparation time: 25 minutes, plus soaking overnight • Cooking time: about 1³/₄ hours

1 cup dried white beans, such as cannellini or navy beans, soaked in cold water overnight

1 large butternut squash, peeled, seeded, and cut into 1-inch cubes

3 tablespoons olive oil

Handful thyme sprigs

1 large onion, sliced fine

1 large clove garlic, minced

14-ounce can diced tomatoes

2 teaspoons tomato paste or sun-dried tomato paste

2¹/₂ cups vegetable or chicken broth

2 tablespoons chopped fresh parsley

Dash of Tabasco sauce

Salt and freshly ground black pepper

1   Drain the soaked beans, cover with plenty of fresh water, and bring to a boil. Boil hard for 10 minutes, then reduce the heat and simmer until tender. This can take anything from 40 minutes to 1¹/₄ hours, depending on the age of the beans. Drain and set aside.

2   While the beans are cooking, preheat the oven to 400°F. Spread the butternut squash cubes out on a heavy baking sheet, sprinkle over the thyme sprigs, rubbing loose some of the leaves as you do so, and drizzle over 2 tablespoons of the oil. Toss well, season with salt, then roast for about 25 minutes, until the squash is tender and lightly browned but still holds its shape.

3   Heat the remaining oil in a large saucepan, add the onion, and cook gently until softened. Stir in the garlic and cook for a few minutes longer, then add the tomatoes, tomato paste, broth, and the drained beans. Bring to a boil, reduce the heat, and simmer for 30 to 40 minutes, until the tomatoes have formed a rich sauce.

4   Stir in the roasted squash and heat through, then add the parsley and a dash of Tabasco. Serve immediately.

NOTE: This soup is suitable for freezing, although the squash might go a little bit mushy.

Parsnip and Gruyère

Soup

The distinctive flavor and texture of parsnips make a rich, thick, and comforting soup. Gruyère is a fine-flavored Swiss cheese, but it works well even without the cheese – instead, add a few tablespoons of chopped parsley.

Serves 4 • Preparation time: 25 minutes • Cooking time: 50 minutes

$1/4$ **stick butter**
1 onion, chopped
1 clove garlic, minced

$1^1/2$ **pounds parsnips, cut into chunks**
$1/2$ **teaspoon ground cumin**
4 cups vegetable or chicken broth

2 slices bacon (optional)
$3/4$ **cup grated Swiss cheese**
Salt and freshly ground black pepper

1   Heat the butter in a large saucepan, add the onion and garlic, and cook gently for a few minutes, until softened.

2   Stir in the parsnips, then cover and cook gently for 10 to 15 minutes, until softened and slightly browned in patches.

3   Stir in the cumin and cook for 1 minute, then add the broth. Bring to a boil and simmer for about 30 minutes, until the parsnips are tender.

4   Meanwhile, if using the bacon, fry it until very crisp, then snip into small pieces. Set aside.

5   Now purée the broth in a blender, return it to the saucepan and season with salt and pepper to taste. Reheat to almost boiling, then remove from the heat and stir in the cheese until melted.

6   Sprinkle the crisp bacon pieces over each bowlful of soup, and serve hot.

NOTE: This soup can be frozen, either before or after adding the cheese (but without the bacon).

Nutritional guidance
Per serving

245 calories
9 g protein
13 g fat (8 g saturated fat)
24 g carbohydrate
8 g fiber
190 mg sodium

✔✔   calcium, phosphorus
✔   vitamin A, folate

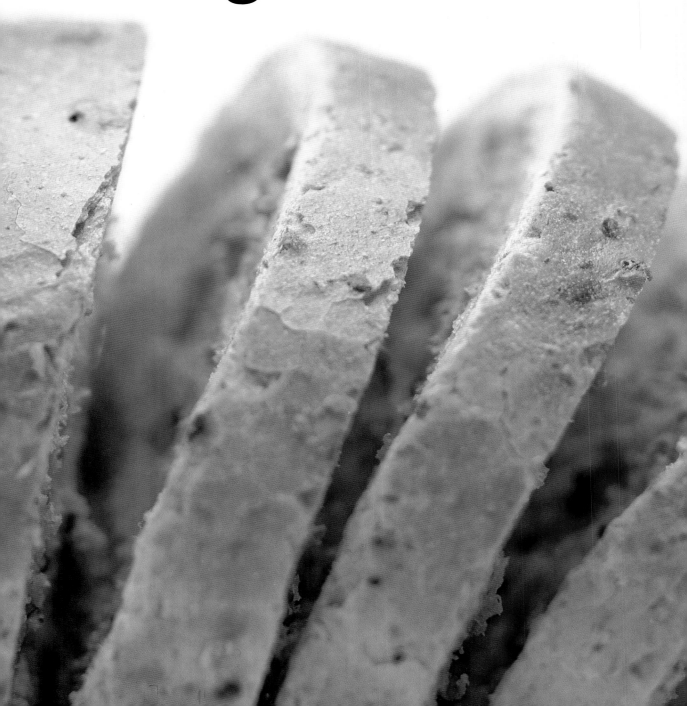

Snacks and
Light meals

Thai-style Vegetable Wrap
with Sweet Chile Sauce

This is a surprisingly filling lunch, and it always makes me feel virtuous to eat so many raw vegetables. It's very good with the sweet chile sauce, but just a sprinkle of a little extra soy sauce is tasty too.

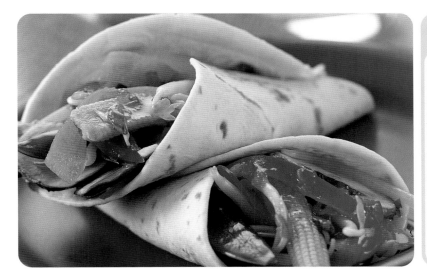

Nutritional guidance
Per serving

213 calories
8 g protein
4 g fat (1 g saturated fat)
37 g carbohydrate
5 g fiber
217 mg sodium

✔✔   vitamin C,
      vitamin A
✔   folate, calcium,
      phosphorus, iron,
      vitamin B6

Serves 2 • Preparation time: 15 minutes • Cooking time: 1 to 2 minutes

½ cup sugar snap peas or snow peas
Large handful bean sprouts
½ cup baby corn, cut lengthwise in half
1 carrot, cut into long shreds on a vegetable peeler

½ red bell pepper, cut into long slivers
4 to 5 mushrooms, sliced thin
2 scallions, halved lengthwise then shredded on the diagonal
2 teaspoons sesame oil
2 teaspoons soy sauce

½ teaspooon Thai fish sauce (*nam pla*)
2 tablespoons cilantro leaves
Two 10-inch tortilla wraps
Sweet chile sauce, to serve

1   Blanch the sugar snap or snow peas, bean sprouts, and corn in a large saucepan of boiling salted water for 1 to 2 minutes, then drain, refresh under cold running water, and drain again. Pat dry on paper towels and put in a bowl with all the other vegetables. Toss with the sesame oil, soy sauce, and fish sauce, then mix in the cilantro leaves.

2   Briefly heat the tortilla wraps, according to the instructions on the package. Put each wrap on a large plate and heap the vegetable mixture down the center of each one.

3   Drizzle with sweet chile sauce, then fold the wrap over into a fan shape or fold in the edges, and roll up. Eat messily with your fingers or rather more elegantly with a knife and fork.

Caponata
with Goat Cheese Toasts

Caponata is more or less the Sicilian answer to ratatouille, incorporating the characteristic sweet and sour flavors of Sicilian cooking and with plenty of celery for a refreshing contrast. The goat cheese toasts make a good accompaniment and add some of that all-important protein. You could also serve the caponata with garlic bread or ciabatta.

Serves 4 • Preparation time: 30 minutes • Cooking time: about 45 minutes

2 small eggplants
Olive oil
2 large onions, chopped
2 red bell peppers, chopped
2 cloves garlic, minced
14-ounce can diced tomatoes
3 to 4 sprigs thyme
6 celery stalks, cut into $^1/_2$-inch thick slices

$^1/_2$ cup black olives
2 tablespoons capers, rinsed and drained
2 tablespoons chopped parsley
6 tablespoons red wine vinegar
About 1$^1/_2$ tablespoons sugar
Salt and freshly ground black pepper

For the goat cheese toasts:
8 slices French bread, cut about $^1/_2$ inch thick
8 slices goat cheese, $^1/_2$ inch thick, cut from a log
Few thyme leaves

1 Cut the eggplants into 1-inch cubes, place in a colander, and sprinkle with salt. Allow to drain for 30 minutes then rinse briefly and pat dry.

2 Meanwhile, heat about 3 tablespoons olive oil in a large skillet, add the onions and red bell peppers and a generous pinch of salt and cook gently for 15 minutes, adding the garlic halfway through.

3 Push the tomatoes through a sieve, or purée them briefly with a hand blender, and add to the skillet with the thyme sprigs. Simmer for 20 minutes.

4 Heat 2 tablespoons olive oil in a separate skillet, add the celery, and fry until lightly colored. Transfer to a plate and set aside.

5 Add some more oil to the skillet and cook the eggplants, in batches, over fairly high heat until lightly browned. Add to the tomato mixture with the celery and cook for 10 to 15 minutes, until the mixture is thick and all the vegetables are tender. Remove from the heat and stir in the olives, capers, and parsley, then add the vinegar and sugar to taste – the flavor should be sweet and sour. Allow to cool to room temperature before serving. (Caponata improves in flavor if left overnight, but don't serve it chilled.)

6 To prepare the goat cheese toasts: Toast the French bread lightly on both sides then top with a slice of goat cheese and sprinkle with thyme leaves. Place under a hot broiler until the cheese begins to melt then serve immediately, on top of the caponata.

Nutritional guidance
Per serving

469 calories
14 g protein
29 g fat (9 g saturated fat)
40 g carbohydrate
7 g fiber
870 mg sodium

✔✔ vitamin C, phosphorus, vitamin A, vitamin E
✔ calcium, iron

Sicilian

Stuffed Peppers

Sicilian cooking is characterized by piquant flavors, hence the combination of dried fruit, mint, capers, and anchovies in the stuffing for these peppers. Served with a green salad, they make a delicious light, summery meal, or you could serve them as an appetizer.

Serves 2 • Preparation time: 25 minutes • Cooking time: 20 minutes

2 large, fleshy red bell peppers
1 cup fresh white bread crumbs
1 tablespoon capers, rinsed and drained
1 tablespoon golden raisins

3 anchovy fillets, chopped fine
1 large clove garlic, chopped fine
2 tablespoons pine nuts, lightly roasted in a dry skillet
1 tablespoon chopped flat-leaf parsley

2 teaspoons chopped mint
About 4 tablespoons olive oil
Salt and freshly ground black pepper

1 Preheat the oven to 350°F.

2 Char the red bell peppers lightly over a gas flame or under a hot broiler; this is just to make the skin easier to remove, so make sure the bell peppers do not become too soft. Leave until cool enough to handle, then peel off the skin and cut the bell peppers in half. Remove the seeds and white ribs, reserving any juices. Place the bell pepper halves in an ovenproof dish in which they fit snugly.

3 Mix together the bread crumbs, capers, golden raisins, anchovies, garlic, pine nuts, and herbs, then add enough olive oil to bind the mixture. Season with salt and pepper.

4 Stuff the pepper halves with this mixture. If the peppers have become very soft and won't hold their shape, you can roll them up around the filling instead. Bake for 15 minutes, until the filling is just beginning to brown, then drizzle over a little olive oil. Return to the oven for 5 minutes. Serve warm or cold.

Nutritional guidance
Per serving

475 calories
8 g protein
34 g fat (4 g saturated fat)
35 g carbohydrate
4 g fiber
324 mg sodium

✔✔ vitamin C,
vitamin A,
vitamin E
✔ phosphorus

English Muffins

with Salsa, Cheese, and Watercress

This very simple idea can be used as a blueprint for all sorts of variations – for example, sharp Cheddar cheese with chutney and lettuce; or, when you're no longer pregnant, forbidden Brie (see page 24) with cranberry sauce and arugula.

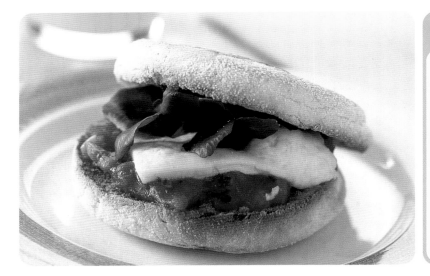

Nutritional guidance
Per serving

302 calories
13.5 g protein
13 g fat (5 g saturated fat)
36 g carbohydrate
2 g fiber
287 mg sodium

✔✔　calcium,
　　　phosphorus
✔　　vitamin A

Serves 2 • Preparation time: 5 minutes • Cooking time: 5 minutes

2 plain English muffins 2 tablespoons salsa	¼ cup mild, crumbly cheese, such as manchego	Handful watercress, thick stalks removed

1　Split the muffins in half and toast them lightly on both sides under the broiler.

2　Spread the bottom halves with the salsa and then cover with the cheese.

3　Return to the broiler for a few minutes, until the cheese is beginning to bubble, then cover with the watercress sprigs, press the tops of the muffins on firmly, and eat immediately.

Croque Monsieur

with Bitter Leaf Salad

The French may not be the greatest fans of fast food but they did invent one of the best quick snacks ever, the Croque Monsieur – a crisp fried ham and cheese sandwich. The name is derived from the French *croquer*, to crunch. Its rich flavors are best complemented by a salad of bitter leaves.

Serves 2 • Preparation time: 10 minutes • Cooking time: 6 to 8 minutes

4 slices brown or white bread
1 cup grated Gruyère cheese
2 slices lean ham, preferably prosciuotto
Dijon mustard

Butter for frying
2 handfuls mixed bitter salad leaves such as endive, frisée, and radicchio
1 tablespoon olive oil

1 teaspoon red wine vinegar
Salt and freshly ground black pepper

1 Cut the crusts off the bread if you prefer, then cover two slices of bread with half the grated cheese. Put the ham on top and spread it with a little mustard, then cover with the remaining cheese. Put the other two slices of bread on top and press the edges together well to seal.

2 Heat a small piece of butter in a skillet until gently sizzling, add the sandwiches, and cook over low to medium heat for 3 to 4 minutes, until golden underneath. Take the sandwiches out of the skillet, add a little more butter to the skillet, then return the sandwiches to the skillet and cook the other side.

3 Meanwhile, put the salad leaves in a bowl, season with salt and pepper, and toss with the oil and vinegar. Divide between two serving plates.

4 Remove the sandwiches from the skillet, cut in half diagonally, and transfer to the serving plates. The melted cheese should be oozing out.

Nutritional guidance
Per serving

482 calories
25 g protein
29 g fat (15 g saturated fat)
33 g carbohydrate
3 g fiber
1033 mg sodium

✔✔ calcium, phosphorus
✔ vitamin A, iron

Focaccia
with Chargrilled Vegetables

A ridged grill pan is useful for this dish but if you don't have one, brush the vegetables with oil and broil them. If you like, you could fill the focaccia with slices of mozzarella or crumbled ricotta as well as the vegetables, or add olives or drained rinsed capers to the dressing.

Serves 2 • Preparation time: 30 minutes • Cooking time: about 15 minutes

2 small red bell peppers
1 eggplant
1 zucchini
1 red onion
Olive oil for brushing

2 tablespoons chopped flat-leaf parsley or basil
1 focaccia loaf, either plain, or flavored with rosemary

For the dressing:
1 clove garlic, minced
3 tablespoons olive oil
1 tablespoon good-quality balsamic vinegar
Salt and freshly ground black pepper

1 Put the red bell peppers under a hot broiler and broil until blackened and blistered all over, turning as necessary. Leave until cool enough to handle, then peel off the skin and discard the seeds. Slice the bell peppers into thick strips, reserving any juices, and set aside.

2 **To prepare the dressing:** Whisk all the ingredients together, adding any juices from the bell peppers.

3 Cut the eggplant and zucchini lengthwise into $1/4$-inch thick slices. Peel the onion and slice that into slightly thicker rounds. Brush the vegetable slices with olive oil and place them on a preheated ridged grill pan, until nicely scored with lines from the grill. Turn and cook the other side. You will have to cook them in batches; when each batch is done, put the vegetables in a shallow dish and drizzle over some of the dressing.

4 When all the vegetables are done, pour over the last of the dressing, stir in the parsley or basil, and, if there is time, allow to marinate for 1 to 2 hours. They are almost as good eaten immediately, though.

5 Wrap the focaccia loaf in foil and heat briefly in a moderate oven so it is just warm. Slice it horizontally in half and sandwich together with the marinated vegetables. Cut into large wedges to eat.

Nutritional guidance
Per serving

642 calories
19 g protein
25 g fat (4 g saturated fat)
88 g carbohydrate
10 g fiber
573 mg sodium

✔✔   vitamin C, vitamin A
✔   calcium, folate, vitamin E, iron

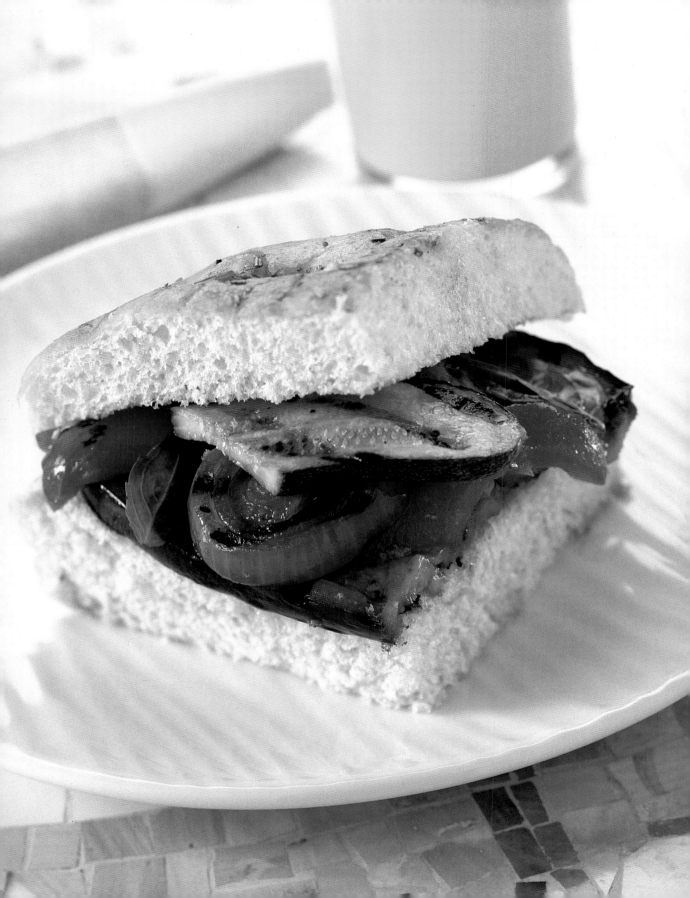

Hummus
with Moroccan Spiced Carrots

The carrots are based on a recipe in Marlena Spieler's wonderful book, *Hot and Spicy*, which anticipated the fashion for fusion food, and is essential reading for chile addicts. Hummus is something you will probably either love or loathe during pregnancy. It came into the latter category for me but some friends got quite a fixation on it. It is certainly very nutritious, rich in protein and vitamins.

Serves 6 • Preparation time: 30 minutes • Cooking time: 20 minutes

15-ounce can garbanzo beans, drained and rinsed
1/3 cup tahini
1 large clove garlic, chopped
4 to 6 tablespoons lemon juice
4 tablespoons olive oil
Generous pinch of cayenne pepper

Salt and freshly ground black pepper
Paprika, to garnish

For the spiced carrots:
1 pound carrots, sliced thin
2 tablespoons olive oil
1 tablespoon white wine vinegar
1 tablespoon lemon juice
1/2 teaspoon ground cumin
1 clove garlic, minced
Pinch of cayenne pepper
1 tablespoon chopped cilantro

1   To prepare the spiced carrots: Boil the carrots until only just tender, then drain thoroughly.

2   Mix together the oil, vinegar, lemon juice, cumin, garlic, cayenne pepper, and a little salt. Pour this dressing over the hot carrots and mix well, then garnish with the chopped cilantro.

3   For the hummus, put all the ingredients except the paprika and seasoning in a food processor, using just 4 tablespoons lemon juice at first. Blend to a grainy purée, then taste and add more lemon juice and cayenne pepper if necessary, plus some salt and pepper. Turn into a serving dish and dust with a little paprika.

4   Serve the carrots, warm or at room temperature, with the hummus and some warmed pita or other Middle Eastern bread. They are also good in whole-wheat rolls.

Nutritional guidance
Per serving

265 calories
6 g protein
21 g fat (3 g saturated fat)
13 g carbohydrate
5 g fiber
110 mg sodium

✔✔   vitamin A
✔   calcium, iron, vitamin C

Pita Bread

stuffed with Falafel, Salad, and Tahini Dressing

These are extremely messy to eat but taste wonderful. Falafel mix or bought falafel make a very acceptable short-cut.

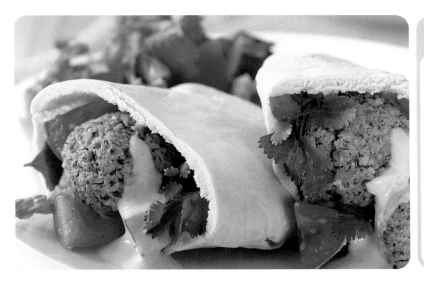

Nutritional guidance
Per serving

375 calories
15 g protein
12 g fat (2 g saturated fat)
56 g carbohydrate
7 g fiber
513 mg sodium

✔✔ phosphorus
✔ calcium, folate,
vitamin C, iron,
vitamin A,
vitamin E

Serves 4 • Preparation time: 25 minutes • Cooking time: 15 minutes

1 cup falafel mix
¹/₂ cucumber, cut into chunks
2 large tomatoes, cut into chunks

2 butter lettuces, shredded
2 tablespoons cilantro leaves
4 pita breads

For the tahini dressing:
4 tablespoons tahini
1 small clove garlic, minced
3 tablespoons lemon juice
Generous pinch of sweet paprika
Salt

1   **To prepare the tahini dressing:** Put the tahini in a bowl, add the garlic and lemon juice, and mix together. Gradually stir in about 2 tablespoons water (the mixture will be lumpy at first but then become smooth again) to obtain a fairly runny sauce. Season with the paprika and salt.

2   Preheat the oven to 375°F. Prepare the falafel mix according to the instructions on the package. Either shape into small rounds or simply drop teaspoonfuls of the mixture onto a lightly greased baking sheet. Bake for about 15 minutes, until cooked through and lightly browned.

3   Meanwhile, mix together the cucumber, tomatoes, lettuce, and cilantro.

4   Put the pita breads on a baking sheet and heat briefly in the oven, until soft, warm, and puffy. Cut each one in half and fill with the falafel and salad, drizzling with the tahini dressing as you go. Serve any leftover salad on the side.

Spinach and Red Bell Pepper

Frittata

Making a flat omelet such as a frittata rather than a French-style omelet ensures that the eggs are thoroughly cooked. It's also a much more versatile dish, just as appetizing served cold as picnic food or part of a packed lunch. To make it more substantial, add a few sliced, boiled, new potatoes to the egg mixture with the spinach and bell pepper.

Serves 4 • Preparation time: 25 minutes • Cooking time: about 15 minutes

1 large red bell pepper
8 ounces baby spinach
2 tablespoons olive oil

1 clove garlic, minced
5 large eggs
¼ cup freshly grated Parmesan

Salt and freshly ground black pepper

1 Roast the red bell pepper under a hot broiler, turning it occasionally, until blistered and blackened all over. Put it in a small bowl, cover, and leave until cool enough to handle, then peel off the skin, discard the seeds, and cut the bell pepper into strips.

2 Discard any large stalks from the spinach, wash the leaves in cold water, and then drain and pat dry.

3 Heat half the oil in a large skillet, add the spinach, then the garlic, and sauté briefly over moderately high heat, turning frequently with a spatula and a wooden spoon, until the spinach has wilted. Season with salt and pepper and then drain in a strainer, pressing out any excess liquid with the back of a wooden spoon.

4 Beat the eggs together in a bowl with some salt and pepper and then stir in the Parmesan, red bell pepper, and spinach.

5 Heat the remaining oil in a 7- to 8-inch heavy-based skillet over high heat. Pour in the egg mixture and immediately reduce the heat to low. Cook gently until the omelet is browned underneath (lift a corner with a palette knife to check) and set nearly all the way through but still a little runny on top.

6 Place the pan under a hot broiler for a few minutes until the omelet is golden, slightly puffed up, and set in the center. Serve warm rather than hot, cut into wedges and accompanied by crusty bread and a green salad or tomato salad.

Nutritional guidance
Per serving

245 calories
16.5 g protein
18.5 g fat (5 g saturated fat)
4 g carbohydrate
2 g fiber
307 mg sodium

✔✔   vitamin A
✔   calcium, folate, vitamin C, vitamin D, iron, vitamin E

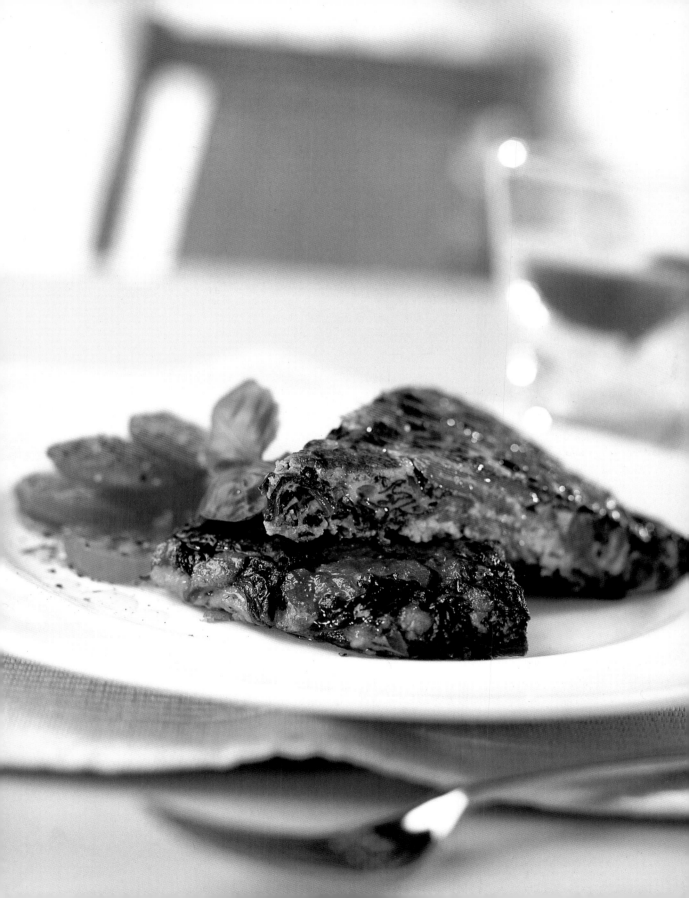

Tuna Pâté on Rye

with Cucumber

This makes much more pâté than you'll need for one snack but it keeps well in the refrigerator. It can also be used to fill hollowed-out tomato halves or as a dip for celery stalks, for a simple hors d'oeuvre or snack.

Serves 2 • Preparation time: 10 minutes

4 slices Scandinavian-style rye bread
Few thin slices cucumber
Paprika for dusting

For the tuna pâté:
7-ounce can good-quality tuna in olive oil, drained
1 cup cream cheese (reduced fat is fine)

2 to 4 teaspoons lemon juice, to taste
2 teaspoons chopped chives
Freshly ground black pepper

1 Put the drained tuna in a bowl with the cream cheese and mix together thoroughly with a fork.

2 Add the lemon juice to taste – the pâté should have a strong lemon flavor – and lots of black pepper, then mix in the chives. Chill lightly.

3 Spread the pâté on the rye bread and cover with cucumber slices. Dust lightly with paprika and serve.

Nutritional guidance
Per serving

434 calories
34 g protein
22 g fat (10 g saturated fat)
27 g carbohydrate
2 g fiber
509 mg sodium

✔✔ vitamin D
✔ vitamin A, iron, vitamin E

Bruschetta

with Tomatoes and Basil

Tomatoes on toast may not sound like a very exciting snack but prepared Italian-style, with perfect, flavorful tomatoes, plenty of good olive oil, and rough, open-textured bread, it is sensational.

Serves 2 • Preparation time: 10 minutes • Cooking time: 5 minutes

8 ounces best-quality ripe tomatoes

Olive oil

About 6 basil leaves, plus a couple of sprigs, to garnish

2 large slices bread from a rustic loaf, such as sourdough

2 cloves garlic, lightly crushed but left whole

Salt and freshly ground black pepper

1 Put the tomatoes in a bowl, pour over boiling water, and leave for 1 minute. Drain, cover with cold water, then drain again. Peel off the skin, cut out the cores, and chop the tomatoes quite fine. Place them in a bowl, drizzle with a little olive oil, then season with salt and pepper. Tear up the basil leaves and mix them in. If the tomatoes are not as flavorful as they should be, add a tiny pinch of sugar or a few drops of balsamic vinegar.

2 Heat a ridged grill pan and toast the bread on it on both sides until it is marked with stripes from the grill. If it gets slightly blackened in places, so much the better.

3 Remove from the grill pan and rub one side of each slice with the garlic cloves.

4 Pour over some olive oil, then top with the tomatoes and sprigs of basil. Eat immediately.

Nutritional guidance
Per serving

139 calories
5 g protein
3 g fat (0.5 g saturated fat)
24 g carbohydrate
3 g fiber
265 mg sodium

✔   vitamin C, phosphorus, vitamin A

Baked Ricotta

with Roasted Tomatoes and Arugula

Baked ricotta has a wonderfully subtle flavor, complemented here by the sweetness of roasted tomatoes and the peppery taste of arugula. It is also full of calcium and protein – essential nutrients during pregnancy – while being fairly low in fat. Both the ricotta and the tomatoes are nicest served lukewarm.

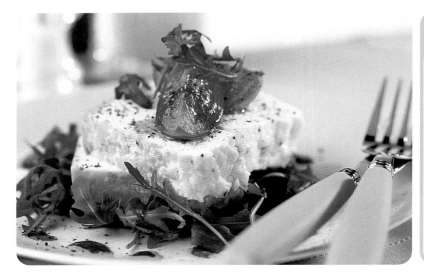

Nutritional guidance
Per serving

263 calories
17 g protein
19 g fat (10 g saturated fat)
7 g carbohydrate
1 g fiber
236 mg sodium

✔✔   calcium,
      phosphorus,
      vitamin A
✔   vitamin C,
      vitamin E

Serves 4 to 6 • Preparation time: 25 minutes • Cooking time: about 2 hours

Butter for greasing the pan
2 tablespoons fine fresh white
   bread crumbs
3 cups ricotta cheese
¼ cup freshly grated Parmesan
2 eggs
1 egg yolk

1 clove garlic, minced
Pinch of freshly grated nutmeg
Salt and freshly ground black
   pepper
2 cups arugula, to serve

For the roasted tomatoes:
6 plum tomatoes
Olive oil
2 teaspoons balsamic vinegar
1 teaspoon sugar

1   **To prepare the roasted tomatoes:** Remove the core from each tomato and cut the tomatoes in half (or into quarters if large). Arrange in a baking pan in a single layer and drizzle with olive oil and balsamic vinegar. Sprinkle over the sugar and some salt and pepper. Bake for about 45 minutes at 275°F until slightly colored and wrinkled. Remove from the oven and keep warm while you prepare the baked ricotta.

2   Increase the oven temperature to 325°F. Generously butter a 1-pound loaf pan and sprinkle it with the bread crumbs, turning to coat it evenly. Tip out any excess crumbs.

3 Put the ricotta cheese in a bowl, add the Parmesan, eggs, egg yolk, garlic, and nutmeg and mix together well. Season generously with salt and pepper. Transfer the mixture to the prepared pan and bake in the oven for about 1 hour 20 minutes, until risen, golden and just firm to the touch. Remove from the oven. Leave the mixture to stand in the pan until lukewarm, then run a knife round the edge, and turn out onto a plate.

4 To serve, cut the ricotta into slices and arrange on serving plates with the roasted tomatoes and a small pile of arugula. Drizzle the syrupy juices from the tomatoes over the cheese and the tomatoes, and drizzle a little olive oil over the ricotta if desired.

Avocado, Tomato, and Cilantro on

Sourdough

This simple sandwich recipe introduces a combination that is really very good indeed. If you have no sourdough bread, multi-grain bread also works well.

Serves 1 • Preparation time: 5 minutes

2 large slices sourdough bread Sweet butter	$1/2$ large ripe avocado, peeled and sliced Lemon juice Few cilantro leaves	1 large tomato, sliced Salt and freshly ground black pepper

1 Spread the bread quite generously with butter and cover one slice with the avocado. Sprinkle with lemon juice and season with salt and pepper.

2 Sprinkle the cilantro on top, then cover with the tomato slices. Season with a little more salt, top with the remaining slice of bread, and eat immediately.

Nutritional guidance
Per serving

585 calories
10 g protein
35 g fat (14 g saturated fat)
61 g carbohydrate
6 g fiber
440 mg sodium

✔✔ vitamin C,
 vitamin A,
 vitamin E
✔ folate, calcium

Salmon and Dill

Quiches

These little quiches make an elegant light lunch or appetizer. The pastry is quick to prepare and the filling is very simple, with no precooking required. If you prefer, use one single 8- to 9-inch tart pan instead of individual pans.

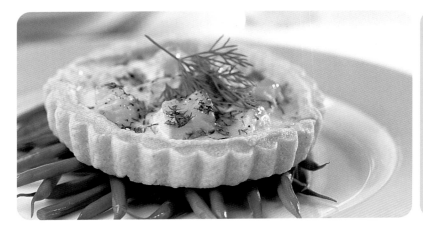

Nutritional guidance
Per serving

868 calories
28 g protein
65 g fat (35 g saturated fat)
46 g carbohydrate
2 g fiber
100 mg sodium

✔✔　vitamin A,
　　　vitamin D,
　　　vitamin E

Serves 4 • Preparation time: 30 minutes, plus chilling • Cooking time: 35 minutes

12 ounces salmon fillet, skinned
1 egg
1 egg yolk
1¼ cups whipping cream

1 tablespoon chopped dill
Salt and freshly ground black pepper

For the pastry:
2 cups all-purpose flour
Pinch of salt
1 stick sweet butter, cut into small cubes
1 egg yolk

1　First make the pastry. Sift the flour and salt into a bowl and rub in the butter with your fingertips until the mixture resembles fine crumbs. Whisk the egg yolk with 2 tablespoons water, add to the flour mixture, and stir together to make a firm but not crumbly dough, adding a little more water if necessary to bind. Wrap in plastic wrap and chill for 1 hour.

2　Preheat the oven to 400°F and place a baking sheet in it to heat up. Roll out the pastry thin and use to line four 4-inch tart pans. Chill for 30 minutes, then line each one with waxed paper, fill with baking beans, and bake blind on the hot baking sheet for 10 minutes, until the pastry looks dry and the paper peels away from it easily. Remove the paper and beans and return the tart cases to the oven for about 5 minutes to bake completely. The pastry should be very lightly colored. Remove from the oven and reduce the temperature to 325°F.

3　For the filling, cut the salmon into ¾-inch cubes and divide them between the pastry cases. Lightly whisk together the egg, egg yolk, cream, and some salt and pepper and pour over the salmon, then sprinkle the chopped dill on top. Bake in the oven for about 20 minutes, until set.

4　Serve warm rather than hot, with a green salad, or steamed snow peas, and new potatoes flavored with chopped mint.

NOTE: The quiches can be frozen.

Potato and Caraway

Latkes

Latkes make a satisfying snack or supper dish. Serve with the traditional accompaniment of apple sauce and sour cream, or with a good tomato chutney or even ketchup.

Serves 4 • Preparation time: 20 minutes • Cooking time: about 15 minutes

1½ pounds potatoes, peeled and grated
1 large clove garlic, minced
2 tablespoons all-purpose flour

1 teaspoon caraway seeds
2 eggs, lightly beaten
2 tablespoons chopped parsley (optional)

Sunflower or peanut oil for frying
Salt and freshly ground black pepper

1 Put the grated potatoes into a large bowl, fill with cold water, and swirl them around a little in order to wash them. Drain well in a large strainer, squeezing out the water with your hands, then place in a clean bowl. Mix in the garlic, flour, caraway, eggs, parsley if using, and some salt and pepper.

2 Heat a thin layer of oil in a large, heavy-based skillet and add tablespoonfuls of the potato mixture, flattening each one with the back of the spoon to give a thin pancake. Fry over medium heat for about 3 minutes each side, until golden and crisp. Drain on paper towels, if necessary, and keep warm while you cook the remaining mixture.

Nutritional guidance
Per serving

304 calories
8 g protein
15 g fat (2 g saturated fat)
37 g carbohydrate
2.5 g fiber
55 mg sodium

✔✔ vitamin E
✔ vitamin C, folate

Quick

Pan Pizza

Don't be put off by the thought of making your own pizza dough. This one contains no yeast and is just about foolproof, besides being very quick to prepare. Two toppings are suggested below (each is enough to serve two), or, if you prefer, make up your own topping. Either way, this is nutritious, colorful, and fast food.

Serves 2 • Preparation time: 30 minutes • Cooking time: about 12 minutes

1²/₃ cups unbleached white bread flour	Salami and mozzarella topping:	Goat cheese and arugula topping:
¹/₂ teaspoon baking powder	12 ounces tomatoes	12 ounces tomatoes
³/₄ teaspoon salt	1 tablespoon olive oil	1 tablespoon olive oil
Freshly ground black pepper	1 clove garlic, chopped fine	1 clove garlic, chopped fine
2 tablespoons olive oil, plus 2 teaspoons for frying	10 wafer-thin slices Italian salami	3 ounces goat cheese, broken into chunks
¹/₂ cup water	5 ounces mozzarella, cut into chunks	14 black olives, used whole
	10 black olives, used whole	2 large handfuls arugula

1   To make the base, put the flour, baking powder, salt, and some black pepper in a bowl and make a well in the center. Mix together the oil and water and pour into the well, then stir together to make a dough, adding a little more liquid as necessary to get a fairly firm but not stiff dough. Turn out onto a work surface and knead for about 5 minutes, until smooth. To knead, simply press the dough out a little with the palm of one hand, fold it in on itself, and give it a quarter turn with the other hand. Place in the bowl, cover with a dishtowel and leave while you prepare the topping (ideally, the dough should be left for 1 hour but this is not essential).

2   For either topping, skin the tomatoes by pouring boiling water over them, leave for 1 minute, then drain and refresh in cold water. Peel off the skins, cut out the cores with a small, sharp knife, and chop the tomatoes fairly fine. Put them in a bowl, add the olive oil, garlic, and some salt and pepper, and toss well.

3   Cut the dough in half, leave one piece covered in the bowl, and roll out the other piece on a lightly floured board to a rough circle about 9 inches in diameter. The dough tends to spring back so it helps if you pull it out by hand a bit too.

4   Brush a large cast-iron skillet or flat griddle with 1 teaspoon olive oil and place over medium-high heat until the heat feels slightly uncomfortable when you hold your hand a few inches above it. Put the circle of dough in the pan and cook for about 3 minutes, until it has brown patches underneath. Turn and cook the other side for about 1 minute, then turn it over again ready for the topping.

5 **To prepare the salami and mozzarella topping:** Spread half the tomatoes over the pizza base, taking them not quite to the edge (if they've given off a lot of liquid, leave most of this behind). Arrange half the salami slices on top, crumpling them a little. Scatter over half the mozzarella. Repeat for a second pizza.

6 Place the pizzas under a very hot broiler until the cheese has melted and the salami is thoroughly heated. Arrange half the olives on top and return to the broiler for 1 minute. Serve, drizzled with a little olive oil and sprinkled with black pepper, if desired.

Nutritional guidance
Per serving

890 calories
37 g protein
49 g fat (17 g saturated fat)
81.5 g carbohydrate
5 g fiber
138 mg sodium

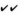 calcium, vitamin A, vitamin E

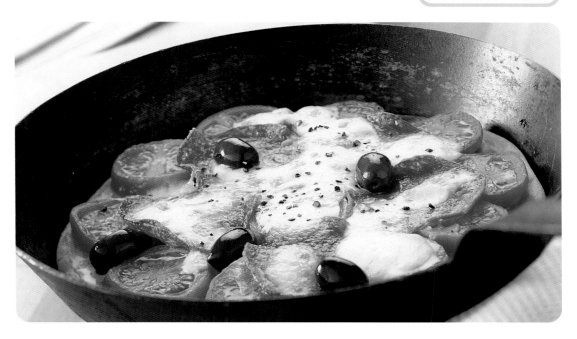

7 **To prepare the goat cheese and arugula topping:** Spread half the tomatoes over the base, then sprinkle half the cheese on top and place under a very hot broiler until the cheese begins to melt. Arrange half the olives on top in a circle, then heap up half the arugula in the center of this. Flash under the broiler for a fraction of a second, just to warm the arugula very slightly, then drizzle with olive oil and serve. Repeat for a second pizza.

NOTE: The base is very crisp at first but will become more pliable after a few minutes.

Nutritional guidance
Per serving

648 calories
18 g protein
30 g fat (7 g saturated fat)
82 g carbohydrate
6 g fiber
786 mg sodium

 vitamin E
✔ calcium, iron vitamin A, vitamin C

Main dishes

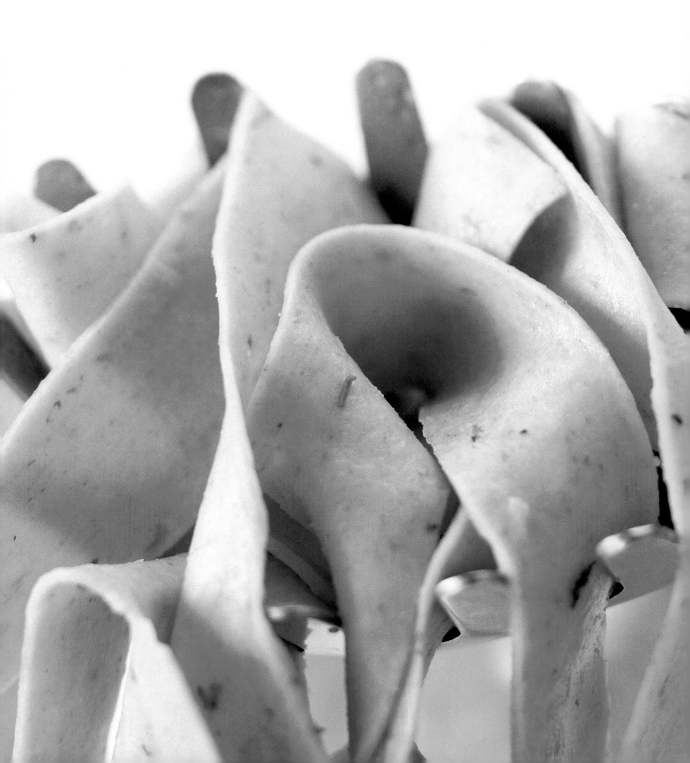

Haddock and Parsley Fishcakes

with Tomato Sauce

The homemade tomato sauce to go with these fishcakes is very good and well worth the effort, because it is so much tastier than store-bought sauce.

Serves 4 • Preparation time: 40 minutes • Cooking time: 50 minutes

1 pound haddock fillet
1 pound potatoes, peeled and cut into chunks
2 anchovy fillets, fine chopped
1 teaspoon mustard
Pinch of cayenne pepper
Grated zest of $1/2$ lemon
2 tablespoons fine chopped parsley

1 small egg, lightly beaten
Flour for dusting
Peanut oil for frying
Salt and freshly ground black pepper

For the tomato sauce:
1 tablespoon olive oil
1 small onion, chopped fine
1 clove garlic, minced
14-ounce can chopped tomatoes
Generous pinch of sugar
1 bay leaf
2 tablespoons heavy cream

1 Put the haddock fillet in a wide shallow pan, cover with water, and bring slowly to a boil. Poach for 2 minutes, then cover, remove from the heat, and allow to cool. Remove the fish from the water and break the flesh into fairly large flakes, discarding the skin and bones.

2 Put the potatoes in a pan of cold salted water, bring to a boil, and simmer until tender. Drain well, return to the pan, and dry over low heat for a minute or so. Mash thoroughly and transfer to a bowl. Mix in the fish and all the remaining ingredients except the flour and peanut oil.

3 With floured hands, shape the mixture into eight cakes, about $3/4$ inch thick. If there is time, chill the fishcakes for an hour or so before frying (they can be prepared up to this stage several hours, or even a day, in advance and kept in the refrigerator).

4 **To prepare the tomato sauce:** Heat the oil in a saucepan, add the onion and garlic, and cook gently until softened. Add the tomatoes, sugar, and bay leaf and simmer for about 20 minutes until well reduced and thickened. Remove the bay leaf, and blend the sauce until smooth, then add the cream and some salt and pepper. Reheat gently.

5 To cook the fishcakes, dust them lightly with flour on both sides. Heat a thin layer of oil in a large skillet and fry the fishcakes over medium heat for about 3 minutes each side, until golden brown. Serve with the sauce.

NOTE: Both fishcakes and sauce can be frozen (freeze the fishcakes at the end of step 3).

Nutritional guidance
Per serving

414 calories
27 g protein
23 g fat (7 g saturated fat)
27 g carbohydrate
3 g fiber
258 mg sodium

✔✔ phosphorus
✔ vitamin A, vitamin E, folate

Marinated Salmon
on Wilted Greens with Ginger, Garlic, and Soy

This is really one of the most delicious ways to cook salmon. Frying it and then transferring it to a hot oven ensures that it has a nicely charred exterior but remains moist inside. If you happen to have a bottle of teriyaki marinade, use that to marinate the salmon – it works just as well.

Serves 2 • Preparation time: 15 minutes • Cooking time: 10 minutes

2 thick salmon fillets, about 6 to 7 ounces each
1 tablespoon peanut oil

For the marinade:
2 tablespoons soy sauce
2 teaspoons sesame oil
$^1/_2$ teaspoon Chinese five-spice powder

For the greens:
1 tablespoon peanut oil
1 large clove garlic, chopped fine
1-inch piece gingerroot, grated
$1^1/_4$ pounds mixed greens, such as bok choy and Chinese cabbage, cut into strips about 3 inches wide
1 tablespoon Shaoxing rice wine
1 teaspoon sugar
2 teaspoons soy sauce
1 teaspoon sesame oil

1 Whisk together all the ingredients for the marinade. Place the salmon fillets in a small, shallow dish, pour over the marinade, and allow to marinate for 1 hour, turning the salmon occasionally and spooning the marinade over it.

2 Preheat the oven to 400°F.

3 Heat the peanut oil in an ovenproof skillet until it is very hot. Add the salmon, skin-side up, and cook for 2 minutes. Turn the salmon skin-side down, transfer to the preheated oven, and cook for 5 minutes. Remove from the oven and allow to stand for 2 to 3 minutes.

4 **To cook the greens:** Heat the oil in a wok or large skillet until very hot, add the garlic and gingerroot, and stir-fry for 1 minute. Add the greens and stir-fry until just wilted, then add the rice wine and sugar and stir-fry for a further minute. Add the soy sauce and sesame oil and toss well. Serve immediately, with the salmon.

Nutritional guidance
Per serving

613 calories
48 g protein
37 g fat (6 g saturated fat)
20 g carbohydrate
4 g fiber
104 mg sodium

✔✔ folate, vitamin D
✔ calcium, iron, vitamin C

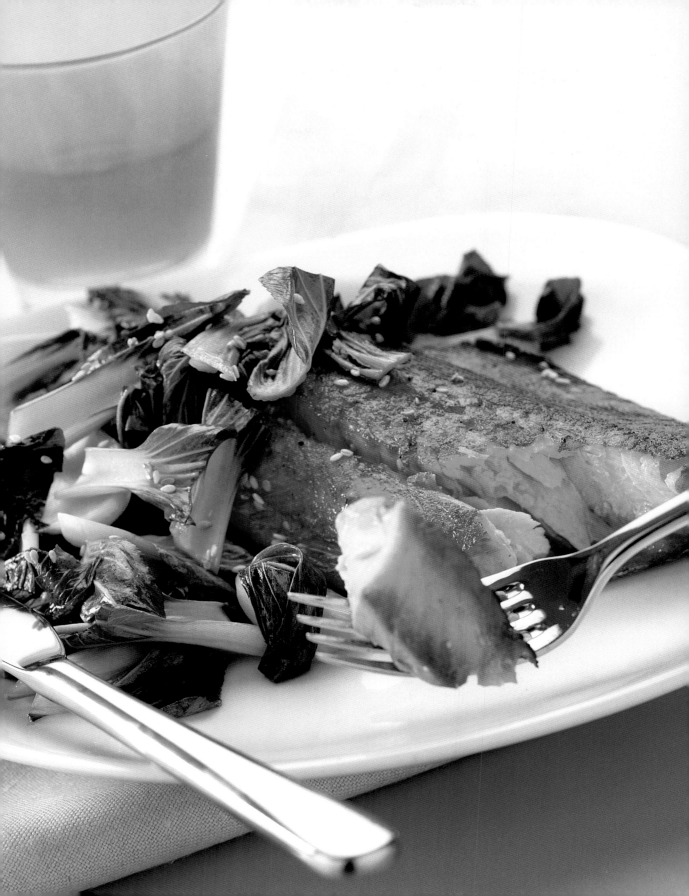

Roast Cod

with Lentils, Red Bell Pepper, and Salsa Verde

Fish and lentils are both useful sources of protein, iron, and folic acid, so together they give you a terrific nutritional boost. The salsa and lentils can be prepared in advance.

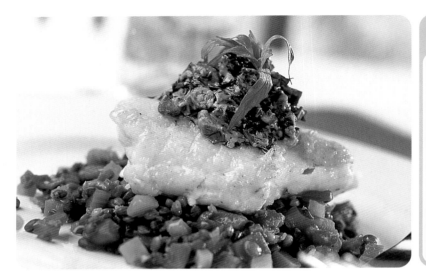

Nutritional guidance
Per serving

500 calories
53 g protein
15 g **fat** (2 g saturated fat)
40 g carbohydrate
7 g fiber
343 mg sodium

✔✔ vitamin C, iron
vitamin A
✔ folate, calcium,
vitamin E

Serves 4 • Preparation time: 30 minutes • Cooking time: 30 minutes

2 tablespoons all-purpose flour
4 thick pieces cod fillet, about 7 ounces each
4 tablespoons olive oil
Salt and freshly ground black pepper

For the salsa verde:
Handful each mint, parsley, and basil leaves
Small handful tarragon leaves (optional)
6 anchovy fillets
1½ tablespoons salted capers, soaked in hot water for 5 minutes, then drained
1 large clove garlic, peeled
1 teaspoon Dijon mustard
Olive oil
Freshly ground black pepper

For the lentils:
1¼ cups French green lentils
1 small carrot, diced very fine
1 celery stalk, diced very fine
1 small onion, diced very fine
1 clove garlic, minced
1 bay leaf
Freshly ground black pepper
1 red bell pepper, roasted, peeled, and chopped fine
Sherry vinegar to taste

1 **To make the salsa verde:** Put the herbs, anchovies, capers, and garlic on a board and chop them very fine (you could do this in a food processor but the texture of the salsa will be more slushy). Put them in a bowl, add the mustard and about 6 tablespoons olive oil, and stir well, mashing everything with the spoon to blend the flavors. Add more olive oil if necessary, so that the sauce has the consistency of thin mayonnaise. Season to taste with black pepper.

2. Put the lentils in a saucepan with the carrot, celery, onion, garlic, and bay leaf, cover with water, and bring to a boil. Simmer for about 20 minutes, until the lentils are tender but still holding their shape, then season with salt and pepper. Stir in the roasted red bell pepper and add a little sherry vinegar, just to brighten the flavors. Keep warm.

3. Preheat the oven to 400°F. Spread the flour out on a large plate and season with salt and pepper. Coat the fish in the flour, dusting off any excess. Heat the oil in a large ovenproof skillet, add the fish, and cook for 2 to 3 minutes each side, until golden brown. Transfer to the oven to roast for 8 to 10 minutes, until cooked through.

4. Divide the lentils between four serving plates, top with the fish, and then spoon a generous amount of salsa verde over that.

Hake

baked on Saffron Potatoes

This is based on a recipe by that remarkably creative chef, Paul Gayler, in his book *A Passion for Potatoes*. He uses whole mackerel instead of hake; if you prefer to use mackerel, increase the cooking time by 5 to 10 minutes.

Serves 2 • Preparation time: 20 minutes • Cooking time: about 40 minutes

3 tablespoons olive oil
1 small red onion, sliced into rings
2 cloves garlic, minced
1/2 teaspoon thyme leaves
1/2 teaspoon oregano leaves

4 plum tomatoes, skinned, seeded, and diced
16 black olives, pitted
12 ounces small new potatoes, peeled and sliced thin
Large pinch of saffron strands

Grated zest and juice of 1 large lemon
2 hake steaks
Salt and freshly ground black pepper

1. Preheat the oven to 375°F.

2. Heat the oil in a large skillet. Add the onion and garlic and fry until softened. Stir in the thyme and oregano, plus the tomatoes and olives. Stir in the potatoes, sprinkle over the saffron, and just cover the potatoes with cold water.

3. Cover and simmer gently for about 15 minutes, until the potatoes are just tender. Season with salt and pepper and stir in the lemon zest.

4. Transfer the mixture to an ovenproof dish. Season the hake steaks and place them on top of the potato mixture. Pour over the lemon juice and bake for 15 to 20 minutes, until the fish is cooked through.

> **Nutritional guidance**
> *Per serving*
>
> 432 calories
> 23 g protein
> 22 g fat (3 g saturated fat)
> 37 g carbohydrate
> 5 g fiber
> 676 mg sodium
>
> ---
>
> ✔✔   vitamin C
> ✔   vitamin A, iron, folate, vitamin E

Chargrilled Lamb
with Ratatouille

The counsel of perfection for ratatouille is to fry each vegetable separately in olive oil but you can make a decent version by frying them all in the same skillet, providing you are careful not to add them all at once. I like to compromise by frying the eggplants separately.

It is worth making double the quantity of this ratatouille. It keeps well in the refrigerator and is good served cold, tossed with pasta, or used as a frittata filling.

Serves 4 • Preparation time: 30 minutes, plus marinating • Cooking time: about 1 hour 10 minutes

2 tablespoons olive oil
1 clove garlic, minced
1 teaspoon thyme leaves
1 teaspoon lemon juice
4 lamb steaks, 7 ounces each
Salt and freshly ground black pepper

For the ratatouille:
Olive oil for frying
2 eggplants, cut into ³/₄-inch chunks
2 onions, diced
2 red bell peppers, cut into ³/₄-inch squares

2 zucchini, cut into ³/₄-inch chunks
2 cloves garlic, minced
3 sprigs oregano or marjoram
14-ounce can diced tomatoes
Small pinch of sugar (optional)

1 Mix together the olive oil, garlic, thyme, lemon juice, and some black pepper. Put the lamb steaks in a shallow dish and rub the oil mixture over them, then cover and set aside to marinate for 1 to 2 hours.

2 **To make the ratatouille**, heat a thin layer of olive oil in a large skillet until it is very hot. Add the eggplant chunks, being careful not to overcrowd the skillet (you may have to cook them in two batches) and reduce the heat a little. Fry until golden all over, turning as necessary. Transfer to a plate, season with salt, and set aside.

3 Heat 2 tablespoons oil in the skillet, add the onions, and cook gently until softened but not colored. Stir in the red bell peppers and cook until softened, then add the zucchini and garlic. Raise the heat slightly, so the zucchini color just a little, and cook until they begin to soften.

4 Return the eggplants to the skillet, add the herb sprigs and canned tomatoes, and season with salt and pepper. Stew slowly, with the skillet half covered, for 20 to 30 minutes, until the vegetables are tender but still hold their shape and the liquid has reduced. Season to taste with salt, pepper, and a pinch of sugar, if needed.

5 To cook the lamb, heat a ridged grill pan until very hot. Put the lamb steaks on it, pressing them down with a spatula, and cook for 3 to 4 minutes, until nicely scored with lines from the grill. Turn and cook for a couple of minutes or so, until cooked through. Transfer to a plate and allow to rest in a warm place for 5 to 10 minutes.

6 Pour any juices from the skillet into the ratatouille. Divide the ratatouille between four serving plates, top with the lamb steaks, and serve.

Nutritional guidance
Per serving

298 calories
19 g protein
17 g fat (2 g saturated fat)
18 g carbohydrate
6 g fiber
47 mg sodium

✔✔ vitamin C, vitamin A
✔ iron, folate

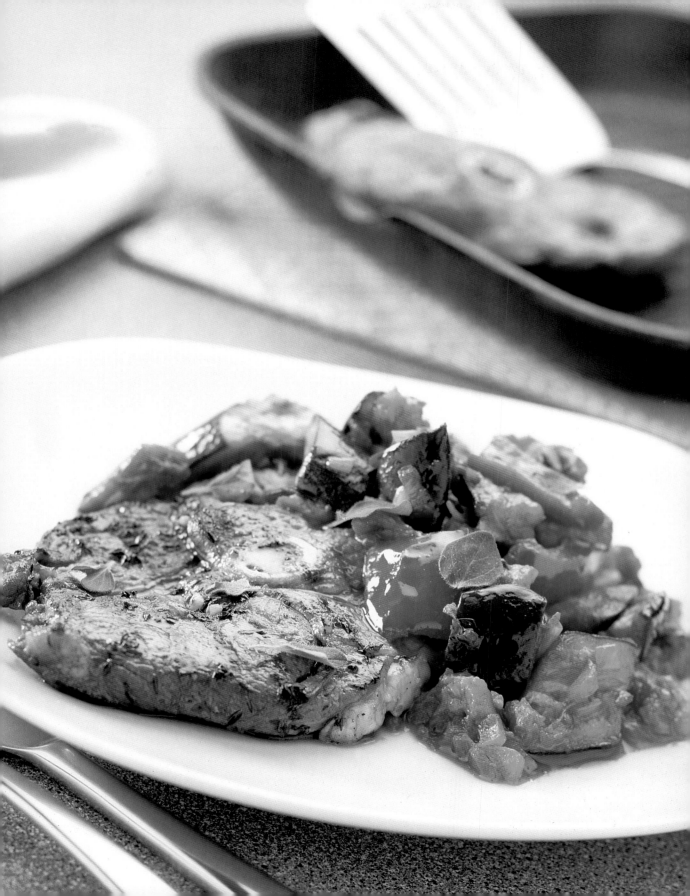

Pork Chops
baked with Fennel, Red Bell Pepper, and Potatoes

In this recipe the meat and vegetables are baked together in the same roasting pan – an easy way to a complete meal. If you do not have time to marinate the chops, it is not essential, although it does make for a better flavor. Simply drizzle them with oil and lemon juice instead and set aside while you prepare the vegetables and heat the oven.

Serves 2 • Preparation time: 30 minutes, plus 2 hours marinating • Cooking time: 40 minutes

2 pork loin chops
1 fennel bulb, trimmed and cut into thick wedges
1 large red onion, peeled and cut into thick wedges
1 large red bell pepper, seeded and sliced thick

8 ounces new potatoes, cut in half
Olive oil
Salt and freshly ground black pepper

For the marinade:
Small bunch thyme
2 cloves garlic, chopped
Grated zest of ½ lemon
2 tablespoons olive oil
1 tablespoon lemon juice

1 Preheat the oven to 425°F.

2 For the marinade, strip the leaves from the thyme and put them in a mortar with the garlic and lemon zest. Pound them with a pestle, together with a small pinch of salt, then gradually stir in the olive oil and lemon juice to make a loose paste.

2 Put the pork chops in a shallow dish and spoon over the marinade, rubbing it into the meat. Cover and allow to marinate for 2 hours.

3 Transfer the chops and their marinade to a roasting pan. Arrange the vegetables over and around them, then drizzle over a little more olive oil, just to moisten them, and season with salt and pepper. Roast in the oven for about 40 minutes, turning once, until the meat is cooked and all the vegetables are tender. Serve immediately.

Nutritional guidance
Per serving

460 calories
43 g protein
17 g fat (4 g saturated fat)
35 g carbohydrate
6 g fiber
107 mg sodium

✔✔ vitamin C, vitamin A
✔ vitamin D, iron, folate

Meatballs

These meatballs are subtly flavored with fennel seed, oregano, and a little paprika but taste satisfyingly rich. Serve them with pasta, rice, or potatoes.

Serves 4 • Preparation time: 40 minutes • Cooking time: 50 minutes

2 slices white crustless bread
Milk
1 small onion, chopped
1 clove garlic, chopped
1 teaspoon fennel seeds
$1/2$ teaspoon dried oregano
1 pound ground pork
$1/4$ teaspoon paprika

1 teaspoon salt
All-purpose flour for dusting
2 tablespoons olive oil
Freshly ground black pepper
Grated Cheddar cheese, to serve
  (optional)

For the tomato sauce:
1 tablespoon olive oil
1 small onion, chopped fine
1 small carrot, shredded
1 clove garlic, minced
3 cups puréed tomatoes
1 bay leaf
2 tablespoons chopped parsley
7-ounce can diced tomatoes

1 Put the bread in a shallow dish and pour over just enough milk to moisten it. Set aside.

2 Put the onion, garlic, fennel seeds, and oregano in a food processor and blend until the onion is chopped fine. Tear up the soaked bread and add it to the food processor with the ground pork, paprika, salt, and plenty of black pepper. Pulse the mixture until just combined (it is important not to overprocess it or the texture of the meat will be affected).

3 Spread out some flour on a large plate. Shape the meat mixture into balls about $1^{1}/_{2}$ inches in diameter, dust them lightly with flour, and then flatten slightly. Heat half the oil in a large skillet, add half the meatballs, and fry over medium heat for about 5 minutes, until browned on both sides. Remove from the skillet and fry the remaining meatballs in the remaining oil in the same way. Set aside.

4 **To prepare the tomato sauce:** Heat the olive oil in a large casserole (ideally, large enough to hold all the meatballs in a single layer), add the onion, carrot, and garlic, and cook gently until softened. Add the puréed tomatoes and bay leaf, season with salt and pepper, and simmer for about 10 minutes, until slightly reduced. Stir in the parsley, then add the meatballs. Pour the diced tomatoes over them, season with a little more salt and pepper, and cook gently for 30 minutes. The meatballs should be done by now but if you are not sure, cut one in half to check.

5 Serve plain or, if preferred, sprinkle a thick layer of grated cheese on top and place under a hot broiler or in a hot oven until browned and bubbling.

NOTE: This dish can be frozen. Freeze the meatballs in their sauce. Reheat gently in a pan after thawing.

Nutritional guidance
Per serving

311 calories
30 g protein
13 g fat (1 g saturated fat)
20 g carbohydrate
3 g fiber
672 mg sodium

✔✔　iron, vitamin B12
✔　　vitamin A,
　　　vitamin C

Quick Chicken
with Pesto and Mozzarella

With its tricolor appearance, this is an attractive way of serving chicken and involves minimum time and effort. Serve with a green vegetable or salad and new potatoes or crusty bread, or in large burger buns with a little shredded lettuce.

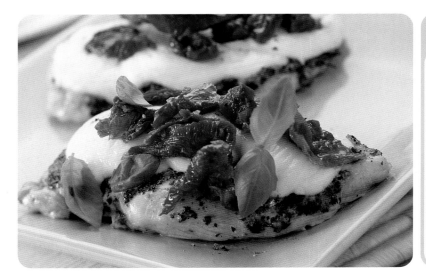

Nutritional guidance
Per serving

636 calories
59 g protein
43 g fat (14 g saturated fat)
2 g carbohydrate
0 g fiber
785 mg sodium

✔✔   calcium, vitamin E, phosphorus
✔   vitamin A, iron, vitamin B2

Serves 2 • Preparation time: 5 minutes • Cooking time: 10 minutes

2 skinless, boneless chicken breasts
Lemon juice

4 tablespoons pesto
4 ounces mozzarella cheese, cut into 6 slices

2 sun-dried tomatoes in oil
Salt and freshly ground black pepper

1   Preheat the oven to 375°F.

2   Put the chicken breasts on a board and pound them out a little with a meat mallet or rolling pin until they are about ½ inch thick. Season both sides with lemon juice, salt, and pepper, then place in a shallow baking pan. Spread the pesto over the top of the chicken and roast in the oven for about 8 minutes, until the chicken is just done.

3   Remove from the oven and increase the temperature to 425°F. Arrange the mozzarella slices on top of the chicken and return to the oven for a few minutes until the cheese has melted. Roughly tear up the sun-dried tomatoes, sprinkle them over the chicken, and serve at once.

Thai Chicken Curry
with Green Beans

Using store-bought green curry paste makes this a quick supper dish. Curry pastes vary quite considerably in strength, so taste yours first to assess the heat level.

Serves 4 • Preparation time: 20 minutes • Cooking time: 30 minutes

2 stalks lemongrass
2 tablespoons peanut oil
2 cloves garlic, chopped fine
2 shallots, sliced fine
1-inch piece gingerroot, chopped fine
2 to 4 tablespoons green curry paste

1 pound skinless, boneless chicken breasts, cut into strips about 2 inches long and 1 inch wide
2 tablespoons Thai fish sauce (*nam pla*)
1 tablespoon sugar
1 tablespoon lime juice

1 teaspoon salt
14-ounce can coconut milk
³/₄ cup green beans, cut in half
1 tablespoon cilantro leaves
1 tablespoon chopped basil

1   Remove the hard outer layers from the lemongrass stalks and chop the tender inner center fine.

2   Heat the peanut oil in a large, deep skillet, add the lemongrass, garlic, shallots, and ginger and fry over medium heat until softened. Add the curry paste (just 2 tablespoonfuls at first, then add more later if necessary) and cook, stirring, for a minute or two.

3   Add the chicken and stir until it is well coated with the curry paste and the flesh has turned white. Stir in the fish sauce, sugar, lime juice, and salt, then add the coconut milk and green beans. Bring to a boil, reduce the heat, and simmer for about 20 minutes, until the chicken is cooked through and the beans are tender.

4   Taste and add more curry paste if necessary, then stir in the cilantro and basil. Serve immediately, with rice.

Nutritional guidance
Per serving

256 calories
29 g protein
10 g fat (2 g saturated fat)
14 g carbohydrate
1 g fiber
662 mg sodium

✔✔   phosphorus, potassium

Perfect

Roast Chicken

For perfect roast chicken you must first buy a decent chicken – organic or very good free range and, less importantly, corn-fed for a good golden color.

Roasting a whole chicken involves about 10 minutes' work but will keep you well supplied with easy meals for several days: the meat can be used in sandwiches, pasta dishes, risottos, or pies. The carcass can be simmered in water with an onion, a carrot, parsley stalks, and a bay leaf, for an hour or so to make a nourishing broth to store in the freezer.

Serves 4 • Preparation time: 10 minutes • Cooking time: 50 minutes to 1 hour

One 3^1/$_4$-pound organic chicken
2 cloves garlic, minced
2 sprigs rosemary
Small handful thyme sprigs

Small handful parsley sprigs, including stalks
2^1/$_2$ tablespoons olive oil
1 lemon

Salt and freshly ground black pepper

1 Preheat the oven to 425°F. Put the chicken in a roasting pan; it should fit snugly. Put the minced garlic and the herb sprigs into the cavity. Spread 1^1/$_2$ tablespoons of olive oil over the chicken and season with salt and pepper. Turn it so it is breast-side down and roast in the oven for 20 minutes.

2 Remove the chicken from the oven and reduce the temperature to 400°F. Turn the chicken breast-side up, squeeze over the juice from the lemon, and drizzle over the remaining olive oil. Sprinkle with a little more salt and return to the oven for 30 to 40 minutes.

3 Check the chicken is cooked through: the legs will be quite loose at the joint if you wiggle them gently, and the juices will run clear when you insert a knife near the thigh bone. Allow to rest for 10 minutes before carving. Serve hot, or allow to cool completely and serve cold.

Nutritional guidance
Per serving (50 g dark meat, 100g light meat)

221 calories
35 g protein
9 g fat (2 g saturated fat)
0.3 g carbohydrate
0.1 g fiber
105 mg sodium

✔✔ niacin
✔   phosphorus

Hungarian-style Beef

Goulash

This is the ideal stew to have simmering on the stove on a cold winter's day, steaming up the kitchen windows and generally gratifying any nesting instincts you might be feeling. Try to buy good-quality paprika for the best flavor. Beef is a rich source of vitamins.

Serves 4 • Preparation time: 25 minutes • Cooking time: about 2^1/$_2$ hours

2 tablespoons peanut oil
1 large onion, sliced
2 large cloves garlic, minced
2^1/$_4$ pounds braising steak, cut into 2-inch pieces
1 tablespoon all-purpose flour
1 tablespoon sweet smoked paprika

^{1}/$_4$ teaspoon hot smoked paprika or pinch of cayenne pepper
1 teaspoon caraway seeds
2 cups meat or vegetable broth
1 green bell pepper, shredded
1 bay leaf
2 teaspoons tomato paste
14-ounce can chopped tomatoes

1 pound potatoes, peeled and diced
3 tablespoons chopped parsley
Salt and freshly ground black pepper

1   Heat half the oil in a large, heavy-based pan, add the onion and garlic, and fry until softened and light browned. Remove from the pan and set aside.

2   Add the remaining oil to the pan and fry the beef, in batches, until the pieces are browned all over. Return the onion and all the meat to the pan. Sprinkle in the flour, paprika, and caraway seeds, and cook, stirring, for 1 minute. Gradually stir in the broth, scraping up any sediment from the base of the pan. Add the bell pepper, bay leaf, tomato paste, and canned tomatoes. Bring to a boil, season with salt and pepper, then cover and simmer very slowly for about 1^1/$_2$ hours, until the meat is tender.

3   Add the diced potatoes and continue to cook for a further 40 minutes or so, until they are tender but still holding their shape. Adjust the seasoning, stir in the parsley.

4   Serve in soup bowls or on deep plates, accompanied by plenty of bread to mop up the delicious, rich gravy.

NOTE: This dish can be frozen.

Nutritional guidance
Per serving

535 calories
60 g protein
19 g fat (2 g saturated fat)
33.5 g carbohydrate
4 g fiber
58 mg sodium

✔✔   vitamin C, iron, vitamin E
✔   vitamin A

Winter Vegetable Casserole
with Horseradish Dumplings

Tabasco and horseradish give this comforting casserole a warm glow. Grated horseradish is available in jars from some supermarkets and delis.

Serves 4 • Preparation time: 30 minutes • Cooking time: $1^1/_4 - 1^1/_2$ hours

1 tablespoon dried mushrooms
3 tablespoons olive oil
$1^1/_2$ cups shallots, peeled but left whole
1 large leek, cut into slices about 1 inch thick
2 cloves garlic, minced
2 parsnips, cut into chunks
2 large carrots, cut into chunks
1 small butternut squash (about 1 pound), peeled, seeded, and cut into chunks

3 to 4 sprigs thyme
2 bay leaves
1 tablespoon all-purpose flour
$1^1/_2$ cups vegetable broth
1 tablespoon tomato paste
2 teaspoons Worcestershire sauce
Generous dash of Tabasco sauce
$1^1/_2$ cups mushrooms, halved
Salt and freshly ground black pepper

For the dumplings:
1 cup all-purpose flour
$1^1/_2$ teaspoons baking powder
$^1/_2$ stick butter, diced
1 cup fresh white bread crumbs
1 tablespoon chopped mixed parsley and chives
2 teaspoons grated horseradish
$^1/_3$ cup milk
Salt and freshly ground black pepper

1 Pour $2^1/_2$ cups boiling water over the dried mushrooms and allow to soak while you prepare the casserole.

2 Preheat the oven to 350°F.

3 Heat 2 tablespoons of the olive oil in a large flameproof pot, add the shallots, and sauté until golden. Add the leek and garlic and sauté until softened. Add the parsnips, carrots, butternut squash, thyme, and bay leaves. Cover and cook gently for 10 minutes, stirring from time to time. Stir in the flour and cook for 1 to 2 minutes, then pour in the mushroom soaking liquid, reserving the mushrooms. Add the broth, tomato paste, Worcestershire sauce, Tabasco, and some salt and pepper and bring to a boil. Cover and transfer to the oven to bake for 25 minutes.

4 Meanwhile, fry the mushrooms in the remaining olive oil until lightly browned. Stir in the reserved dried mushrooms, season with salt, and set aside.

5 **To prepare the dumplings:** Sift the flour and baking powder into a bowl and rub in the butter with your fingertips until the mixture resembles crumbs. Stir in the bread crumbs, herbs, and some seasoning. Mix the horseradish with the milk and then gradually add it to the flour mixture to give a soft, but not sticky, dough. With lightly floured hands, shape into eight to ten dumplings.

6 Remove the pot from the oven, taste the liquid, and season with more salt, pepper, Worcestershire sauce, or Tabasco, as necessary. Stir in the mushrooms.

7 Arrange the dumplings on top of the vegetables and return the pot to the oven, uncovered, for 25 to 30 minutes to cook the dumplings. Serve with lots of mashed potatoes (pages 112-113).

NOTE: This dish can be frozen (but not the dumplings).

Nutritional guidance
Per serving

402 calories
10 g protein
20 g fat (6 g saturated fat)
50 g carbohydrate
10 g fiber
203 mg sodium

✔✔   vitamin A
✔   calcium, folate, vitamin C, iron

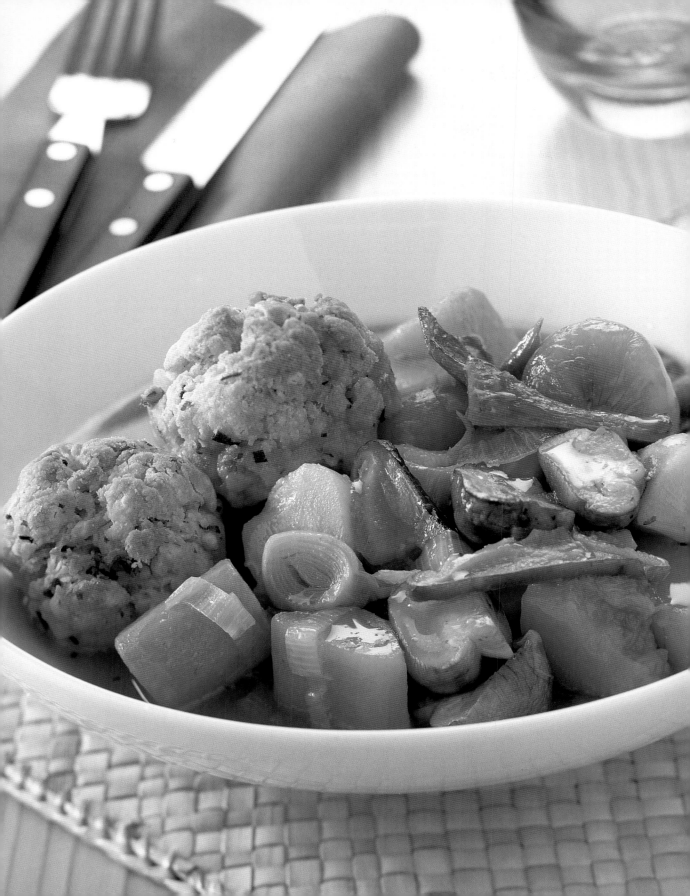

Seven-Vegetable
Couscous

In some parts of North Africa it is considered lucky to include seven vegetables in your couscous. The stew is usually made with meat as well, such as lamb or chicken, but this vegetable version has so much flavor it hardly seems necessary to add anything else.

Serves 4 • Preparation time: 30 minutes • Cooking time: 1 hour

3 tablespoons olive oil
1 large onion, chopped
2 cloves garlic, chopped fine
2 teaspoons ground cumin
1 teaspoon ground coriander
$^1/_2$ teaspoon ground cinnamon
Large pinch of hot red pepper flakes
8 ounces potatoes, cut into chunks
1 sweet potato, about 10 ounces, cut into chunks
4 carrots, cut into chunks
14-ounce can tomatoes
4 cups chicken or vegetable broth

2 small turnips, cut into quarters
3 small zucchini, cut into chunks
$^3/_4$ cup green beans, cut in half
15-ounce can garbanzo beans, drained and rinsed
1 to 2 teaspoons harissa paste, (North African spice)
2 teaspoons lemon juice
4 tablespoons rough chopped cilantro leaves
1 tablespoon chopped mint (optional)
Salt and freshly ground black pepper

For the couscous:
$1^1/_4$ cups couscous
$^1/_3$ cup raisins
1 tablespoon butter
Large pinch of saffron
$1^1/_2$ cups boiling water

1 Heat the oil in a large saucepan, add the onion and garlic, and fry until softened and lightly browned. Stir in the cumin, coriander, cinnamon, and hot red pepper flakes and cook for 1 minute, then stir in the potatoes, sweet potato, and carrots. Add the tomatoes and broth, bring to a boil, and simmer for about 20 minutes, until the vegetables are almost tender.

2 Add the turnips and cook for a further 10 minutes, then add the zucchini, green beans, and half the drained garbanzo beans. Simmer for about 20 minutes, until all the vegetables are tender.

3 Meanwhile, prepare the couscous. Put the couscous in a bowl with the raisins and the remaining garbanzo beans and dot the butter over the top. Mix the saffron with the boiling water, add some salt and pepper, and pour it over the couscous. Cover and allow to stand for 15 minutes. Fluff up the couscous with a fork, using your fingers to break up any lumps if necessary.

4 Season the stew with salt and pepper, then remove $^2/_3$ cup of the liquid and put it in a small bowl. Stir in the harissa paste, followed by the lemon juice and 1 tablespoon cilantro leaves to make a spicy sauce. Stir the remaining cilantro into the vegetable stew, with the mint, if using.

5 Transfer the couscous to a large platter and mound it up. Spoon some of the vegetables on top. Serve with the remaining vegetable stew and the spicy sauce, together with some extra harissa on the side for those who like it really spicy.

Nutritional guidance
Per serving

557 calories
15 g protein
15 g fat (4 g saturated fat)
95 g carbohydrate
11.5 g fiber
294 mg sodium

✔✔ vitamin A, vitamin C, vitamin E
✔ calcium, iron, folate

Brown Rice

with Celery and Parmesan

This combines the clean, refreshing taste of celery with nutty brown rice. It is a perfect choice for tired tastebuds or for those occasions when you don't feel up to eating anything too elaborate.

Arborio (risotto) rice can be used instead of brown rice to make a shortcut risotto, in which case you will need to increase the broth quantity by $2/3$ cup, and reduce the cooking time by 20 minutes. You could also substitute leeks for the celery and stir in a handful of frozen peas toward the end.

Serves 2 • Preparation time: 15 minutes • Cooking time: 45 minutes

1 tablespoon olive oil
4 celery stalks, including a few leaves if possible, sliced fine
1 clove garlic, minced
1 cup brown rice

$2^1/_2$ cups vegetable or chicken broth
2 to 3 tablespoons fine chopped parsley

$1/_4$ cup freshly grated Parmesan, plus extra to serve
Salt and freshly ground black pepper

1 Heat the olive oil in a heavy-based saucepan, add the celery and garlic, then cover and cook gently for about 10 minutes, until the celery is beginning to soften.

2 Stir in the rice, then pour in the broth and bring to a boil. Reduce the heat, cover, and simmer for about 35 minutes, until the rice is tender and most of the liquid has been absorbed. It should be quite moist, so add a little more broth or water if necessary.

3 Stir in the parsley and some salt and pepper, then remove from the heat and stir in the grated Parmesan. Serve sprinkled with some extra Parmesan.

Nutritional guidance
Per serving

470 calories
12 g protein
13 g fat (4 g saturated fat)
82 g carbohydrate
3 g fiber
177 mg sodium

✔✔ phosphorus
✔ calcium, iron, vitamin E

Penne

with Broccoli, Anchovies, and Chile

I like to cook the broccoli until it is soft, so it starts to disintegrate and form a sauce for the pasta. The quantities given for the garlic, anchovies, and red hot pepper flakes are just a suggestion – vary them according to your taste.

Serves 2 • Preparation time: 10 minutes • Cooking time: about 20 minutes

3 cups broccoli florets
7 ounces pasta shapes, such as penne
3 tablespoons olive oil
1 large clove garlic, minced

Generous pinch of red hot pepper flakes
4 anchovy fillets, chopped
1 tablespoon halved black olives (optional)

3 tablespoons freshly grated Parmesan, plus extra to serve
Salt and freshly ground black pepper

1 Boil or steam the broccoli until it is tender, then drain well.

2 Cook the pasta in a large saucepan of boiling salted water for 8 to 10 minutes, until *al dente*.

3 Meanwhile, heat the olive oil in a large skillet, add the garlic and hot red pepper flakes, and cook gently for a couple of minutes, until the garlic releases its aroma. Add the anchovies and cook, stirring, until they begin to disintegrate into the oil and form a sauce. Add the broccoli and 1 tablespoon water from the pasta saucepan and cook, stirring, over slightly higher heat, until the water has evaporated and the broccoli has started to break up. Add the olives, if using, then season with a little salt and plenty of pepper.

4 Drain the pasta, add it to the sauce with the grated Parmesan, and mix well. Adjust the seasoning and serve immediately, with extra cheese.

Nutritional guidance
Per serving

608 calories
24 g protein
25 g fat (5.5 g saturated fat)
78 g carbohydrate
6 g fiber
392 mg sodium

✔✔ vitamin C
✔ calcium, iron, folate, vitamin A, vitamin E

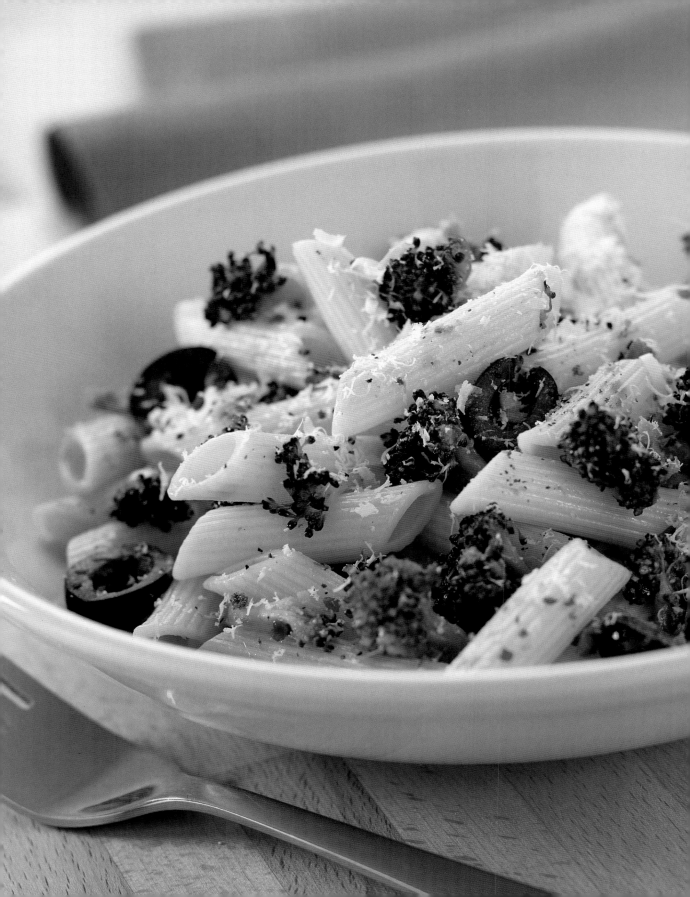

Butternut Squash Ravioli
with Sage and Lemon Butter

If you enjoy spending a leisurely afternoon in the kitchen occasionally, do try out this recipe. These lovely golden ravioli are not difficult to make – in fact they're child's play – but they do take a little time. If you prefer not to make your own pasta, you could use wonton wrappers instead.

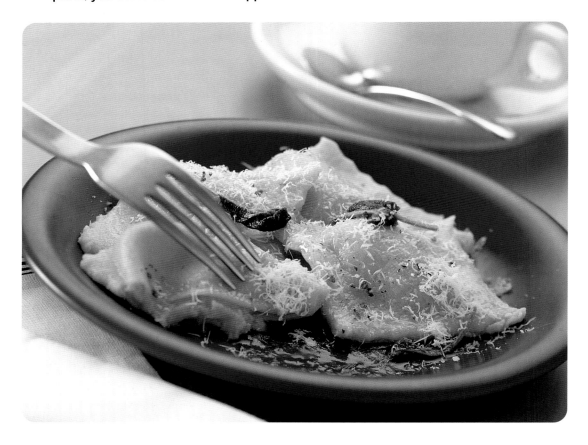

Serves 4 • Preparation time: 1¹/₂ to 2 hours • Cooking time: 1 hour

3 eggs
¹/₂ cup semolina (if unavailable use an extra ¹/₂ cup flour)
2¹/₂ cups unbleached white bread flour

For the filling:
1 small butternut squash
¹/₂ cup freshly grated Parmesan, plus extra to serve
¹/₂ cup fresh white bread crumbs
Pinch of freshly grated nutmeg
Pinch of ground ginger
Grated zest of 1 lemon
1 egg yolk

1 teaspoon water
Salt and freshly ground black pepper

For the sage and lemon butter:
¹/₂ stick unsalted butter
About 12 sage leaves
Lemon juice

1   Preheat the oven to 400°F.

2   For the filling, cut the butternut squash in half, remove the seeds, then wrap each half in a piece of lightly oiled foil and bake in an oven for about 45 minutes, until tender.

3   Meanwhile, make the pasta. Put the eggs, semolina, and 2 cups of the flour into a food processor and blend until it forms a ball. Check the texture: if it is soft and sticky, blend in the remaining flour a little at a time until you achieve the right consistency – it should be firm, but not stiff, and only very slightly sticky. Turn out onto a floured work surface and knead for 1 to 2 minutes, until smooth. If the dough feels too stiff, return it to the food processor and mix in 1 to 3 teaspoons water; if too soft, add a little more flour. Wrap the dough in plastic wrap and leave in the refrigerator for 1 hour. This is not absolutely essential, so don't worry if you don't have time.

> **Nutritional guidance**
> *Per serving*
>
> 581 calories
> 23 g protein
> 22 g fat (11 g saturated fat)
> 77 g carbohydrate
> 4 g fiber
> 277 mg sodium
>
> ---
>
> ✔✔   vitamin A, calcium
> ✔   iron, vitamin D, vitamin C

4   When the butternut squash is cool enough to handle, scrape out the flesh. You will need 1¼ cups. Put this in the food processor with all the remaining filling ingredients and blend until smooth. Chill for 30 minutes, if you have time, to make it easier to handle.

5   Cut the pasta dough in half, return one piece to the refrigerator, and roll out the other on a lightly floured work surface. You have to roll it into a paper-thin sheet, so that you can almost see through it. Don't worry; if the dough has the correct consistency it's very tough and stretchy and is unlikely to tear.

6   When you have a large rectangle, trim the edges and then fold it in half to find the center. Make a small nick at each side where the center point is, then unfold the dough. Cover one half with ½ teaspoonfuls of filling, placed about 1 inch apart, in neat rows. Brush lightly between the rows with water, using a pastry brush, then fold over the other half of the dough. Gently press down around each mound of filling with your fingers to ensure there are no air pockets. Cut between the mounds with a ravioli cutter (a little wheel with a fluted edge) or with a sharp knife, making sure the edges are well sealed.

7   Place the ravioli on a tray sprinkled with semolina (or flour), and cover with a dishtowel, while you roll out and fill the remaining dough in the same way. The ravioli can be kept at room temperature for a couple of hours or in the refrigerator for up to 8 hours – any longer and they start to discolor.

8   **To prepare the sage and lemon butter:** Heat the butter in a small saucepan until frothy then add the sage leaves, a generous squeeze of lemon juice, and some salt and pepper. Set aside.

9   Cook the ravioli in a large saucepan of boiling salted water for about 3 minutes, until just tender, then drain well and divide between four warm serving plates. Quickly reheat the butter and pour it over the pasta, making sure each plateful gets a few sage leaves. Serve immediately, with grated Parmesan.

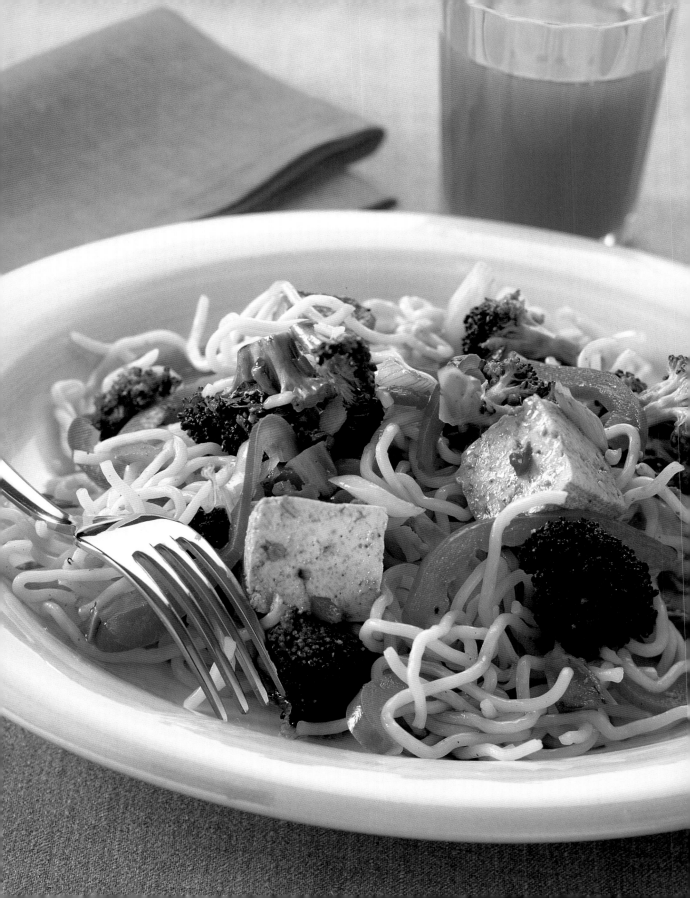

Buckwheat Noodles

with Tofu and Broccoli

You could use any noodles for this but I like the earthiness of buckwheat with the broccoli and tofu.

Serves 2 • Preparation time: 20 minutes • Cooking time: about 15 minutes

5 ounces firm tofu (bean curd), cut into cubes

8 ounces broccoli

6 ounces buckwheat (soba) noodles

2 tablespoons peanut oil

2 cloves garlic, chopped fine

2-inch piece gingerroot, chopped fine

1 red chile, chopped fine

4 scallions, sliced

1/2 red bell pepper, cut into long slivers

1 tablespoon soy sauce

2 teaspoons rice wine vinegar

For the marinade:

1 tablespoon peanut oil

1 tablespoon soy sauce

1 teaspoon honey

1/2 teaspoon Chinese five-spice powder

1 clove garlic, minced

1 Mix all the ingredients for the marinade together in a small shallow bowl. Add the tofu cubes and allow to marinate, turning occasionally, while you prepare the rest of the ingredients.

2 Divide the broccoli into small florets. Peel the stalks and slice them on the diagonal. Cook the noodles according to the instructions on the package and drain.

3 Heat the oil in a wok or large skillet, add the garlic, ginger, and red chile, and stir-fry over fairly high heat for 1 to 2 minutes. Add the broccoli florets and stalks, the scallions, and red bell pepper, and stir-fry until the broccoli is beginning to soften. Add the noodles, the tofu and its marinade, and 3 tablespoons water. Mix well, then add the soy sauce and rice wine vinegar. Mix again, cook for a further minute or two, and serve.

Nutritional guidance
Per serving

607 calories
20 g protein
22 g fat (4 g saturated fat)
86 g carbohydrate
6 g fiber
18 mg sodium

✔✔ calcium, iron, vitamin C, vitamin A

✔ folate

Pasta
with Smoked Bacon and Cabbage

Pasta and cabbage make a healthy combination and this is one of the nicest ways to eat cabbage I know. A good dish to eat on a cold day.

Serves 2 • Preparation time: 15 minutes • Cooking time: 20 minutes

1 small green cabbage (about 1¼ pounds), chopped (central core removed)

3 slices bacon, cut into small strips
1 clove garlic, minced
1 tablespoon olive oil (optional)

7 ounces penne or other pasta shapes
½ cup freshly grated pecorino romano or Parmesan

1 Cook the cabbage in 1 inch of boiling, salted water until just tender, about 5 minutes, then drain well.

2 Gently cook the bacon in a large skillet until it releases its fat, then add the garlic and the olive oil, if needed. Raise the heat a little and fry until the garlic becomes aromatic and the bacon is browned. Add the cabbage and toss together well until the cabbage is thoroughly heated.

3 Cook the pasta in a large saucepan of boiling salted water until tender but still firm, then drain. Return it to the saucepan, season with salt and pepper, and mix with half the cheese. Mix in the cabbage and bacon and then the remaining cheese. Adjust the seasoning (you may need more pepper) and serve immediately.

Nutritional guidance
Per serving

591 calories
34 g protein
14 g fat (7 g saturated fat)
88 g carbohydrate
10 g fiber
804 mg sodium

✔✔ calcium, folate, vitamin C, vitamin A
✔ iron, vitamin B12

Baked Rigatoni
with Spinach and Mushrooms

If you're yearning for comfort food this is just the dish. Spinach and mushrooms prevent it being too rich. Try to choose a good, mature, well-flavored hard cheese for the sauce, otherwise it will be bland – although you could always improve the flavor with a teaspoon or so of mustard if you like. If you are making this for two, put half of it in a separate dish and freeze it. This sort of filling, wholesome food is ideal to store in the freezer for those busy days just after your baby is born.

Serves 4 • Preparation time: 40 minutes • Cooking time: about 50 minutes

12 ounces fresh young spinach
2 tablespoons olive oil
Freshly grated nutmeg
Piece of butter
2$^1/_2$ cups mushrooms, cut into
    chunks
1 clove garlic, minced

8 ounces rigatoni or penne
Salt and freshly ground black
    pepper

For the cheese sauce:
3 tablespoons butter
$^1/_3$ cup all-purpose flour
2$^1/_2$ cups warm milk
1 cup mature hard cheese, such
    as Cheddar, grated
Squeeze of lemon juice

1 Remove any large stalks from the spinach, wash the leaves, and drain in a colander.

2 Heat half the olive oil in a large skillet, add the spinach, and sauté briefly until wilted, turning the spinach over with 2 wooden spoons if necessary so it cooks evenly. Season with salt, pepper, and nutmeg and set aside.

3 Heat the remaining oil and the butter in a large skillet, add the mushrooms, and sauté over fairly high heat until tender and lightly browned, tossing in the garlic and seasoning with salt and pepper 1 to 2 minutes before they are done. Remove from the heat and set aside.

4 To make the sauce, melt the butter in a saucepan, stir in the flour, and cook, stirring, for 2 minutes. Add the warm milk a little at a time, stirring constantly, then bring to a boil, stirring until the sauce thickens. Cook for about 5 minutes over very low heat, then remove from the heat and stir in the cheese until melted. Season with salt, pepper, and a small squeeze of lemon juice.

5 Cook the pasta in a large saucepan of boiling salted water until tender but still firm, then drain. Stir in a few tablespoons of the sauce, followed by the mushrooms and spinach, then turn into a shallow dish about 8 inches square. Pour over the remaining sauce and bake in an oven preheated to 400°F for about 20 minutes, until browned and bubbling.

NOTE: This dish can be frozen (freeze before baking).

Nutritional guidance
Per serving

615 calories
26 g protein
32 g fat (17 g saturated fat)
60 g carbohydrate
5 g fiber
548 mg sodium

✔✔   calcium, folate,
       vitamin A
✔   iron, vitamin C

Accompaniments

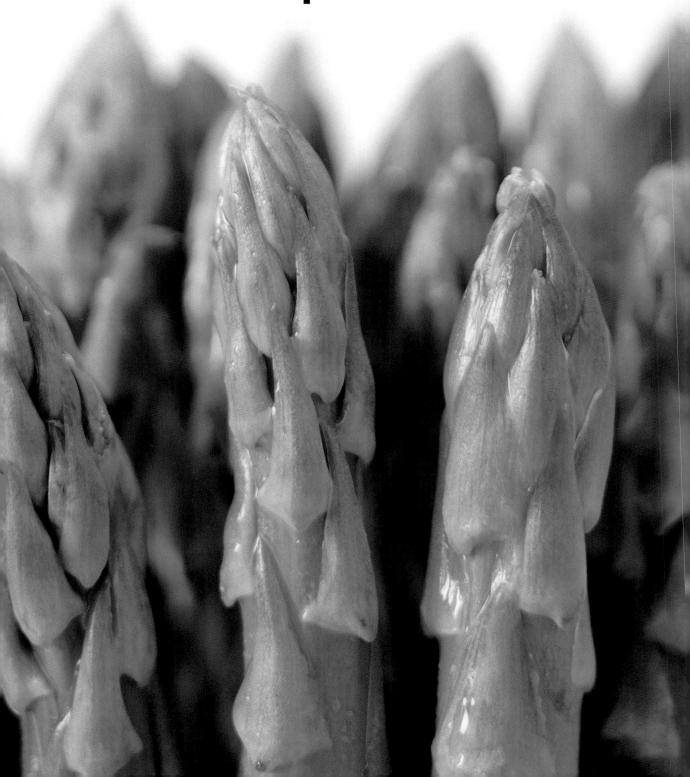

Honey-roasted Carrots
with Thyme

Carrots deserve to be given special treatment occasionally. These take no longer to prepare than boiled carrots and are a rather virtuous way of satisfying a sweet tooth.

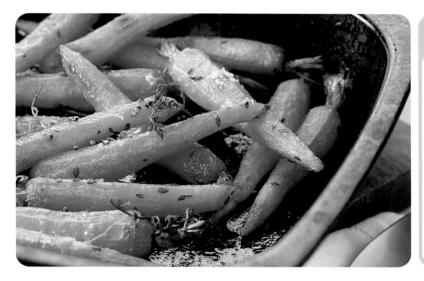

Nutritional guidance
Per serving

166 calories
1 g protein
12 g fat (4 g saturated fat)
14 g carbohydrate
4 g fiber
71 mg sodium

✔✔ vitamin A
✔   vitamin E

Serves 2 • Preparation time: 10 minutes • Cooking time: 30 to 40 minutes

2 tablespoons olive oil
12 ounces long, slender, young carrots, peeled

Small bunch thyme, preferably lemon thyme
1 teaspoon honey

Salt and freshly ground black pepper

1 Heat the oven to 400°F.

2 Pour the olive oil into a small roasting pan and heat briefly in the oven. Add the carrots and roll them around to coat with the oil, then add the thyme and a sprinkling of salt. Roast for about 20 minutes, until lightly browned and almost tender.

3 Drizzle the carrots with the honey (this is easier if you heat the teaspoon first), mix well, and then return to the oven for 10 to 20 minutes, until the carrots are tender and lightly caramelized.

Three Great Mashes

These wonderfully hearty mashes go well with ham, sausages, or ratatouille and other vegetables. The luminous orange of the sweet potato and chile mash is excellent with broiled fish.

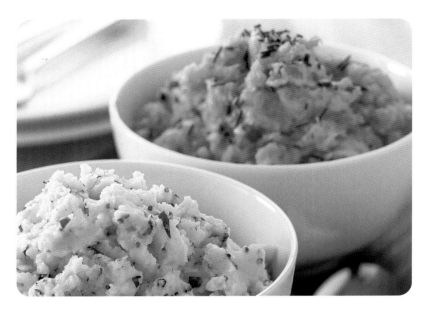

Cheese and Mustard Mash

Serves 2 • Preparation time: 20 minutes • Cooking time: 25 minutes

1 pound potatoes, peeled and cut into chunks
6 tablespoons milk
1 tablespoon butter

2 teaspoons mustard
³/₄ cup grated sharp Cheddar cheese

1 tablespoon chopped parsley
Salt and freshly ground black pepper

1. Put the potatoes in a saucepan of cold salted water, bring to a boil, and simmer until tender. Drain well, then return to the saucepan and dry over low heat for a few seconds.

2. Add the milk and butter and mash well, then beat in the mustard, followed by the cheese and the parsley. Season to taste with salt and pepper, and serve at once.

Nutritional guidance
Per serving

406 calories
16 g protein
21 g fat (13 g saturated fat)
41 g carbohydrate
3 g fiber
495 mg sodium

✔✔ calcium, folate, vitamin A
✔ vitamin C

Sweet Potato and Chile Mash

Serves 2 • Preparation time: 15 minutes • Cooking time: about 1 hour

About 1½ pounds orange-fleshed sweet potatoes
1 tablespoon olive oil
1 small onion, diced fine
1 clove garlic, minced

½ to 1 fresh red chile, to taste, seeded and chopped fine
¼ cup cream cheese (reduced fat is fine)
Freshly grated nutmeg

Squeeze of lime or lemon juice
2 teaspoons chopped chives
Salt and freshly ground black pepper

1 Preheat the oven to 400°F. Prick the potatoes with a fork and then bake for 1 hour until tender.

2 Meanwhile, heat the olive oil in a small skillet, add the onion, garlic, and chile, and fry gently until the onion is soft and lightly browned.

3 When the potatoes are done, peel off the skin and put the flesh into a saucepan. Add the cream cheese and mash well, then stir in the onion mixture. Season to taste with nutmeg, lime or lemon juice, salt, and plenty of black pepper. Beat with a wooden spoon until creamy (do this over low heat if the potatoes are getting cold).

4 Stir in the chives and serve immediately.

Nutritional guidance
Per serving

401 calories
7 g protein
10 g fat (3 g saturated fat)
75 g carbohydrate
9 g fiber
136 mg sodium

✔✔ vitamin C, vitamin A, vitamin E
✔ phosphorus, iron

Potato and Celeriac Mash

Serves 2 • Preparation time: 20 minutes • Cooking time: about 25 minutes

1 small celeriac, about 12 ounces to 1 pound
8 ounces potatoes, peeled and cut into chunks

2 cloves garlic, peeled
¼ stick butter
2 tablespoons milk or light cream

Salt and freshly ground black pepper

1 Peel the celeriac, removing all the tough bits of skin and rubbing it with lemon juice if it starts to discolor. Cut it into chunks, then put it in a saucepan of cold salted water with the potatoes and garlic cloves and bring to a boil. Reduce the heat and simmer until tender.

2 Drain well and push the vegetables through a strainer, or a potato ricer if you have one, into a clean saucepan. Over low heat, beat in the butter and milk or cream, then season to taste with salt and pepper.

Nutritional guidance
Per serving

213 calories
5 g protein
11 g fat (7 g saturated fat)
24 g carbohydrate
7 g fiber
246 mg sodium

✔ folate, vitamin A, iron, vitamin C

Gratin

Dauphinois

There is no point skimping on the cream and butter in this unashamedly luxurious dish. It *is* rich, it *is* high in fat, and eaten once in a while it won't do you any harm at all and will make you feel rather pampered. Besides, potatoes are an important source of vitamin C, and cream contains vitamin A, calcium and protein, so it's not a nutritionally empty treat.

Serves 4 • Preparation time: 15 minutes • Cooking time: $1^3/_4$ hours

$^1/_4$ stick butter
$1^3/_4$ pounds potatoes

$1^1/_4$ cups whipping cream
1 clove garlic, minced
Freshly grated nutmeg

Salt and freshly ground black pepper

1 Preheat the oven to 300°F.

2 Smear the butter liberally over the base and sides of an 8-inch gratin dish. Peel the potatoes and slice them thin. This is easily done with the slicing attachment of a food processor or a mandolin but you could do it by hand with a large sharp knife. Arrange them in the dish, seasoning with salt and pepper between the layers and making a neat top layer of overlapping slices.

3 Put the cream, garlic, some nutmeg, salt, and pepper in a saucepan and bring just to a boil.

4 Pour this mixture over the potatoes, adding it slowly so it filters in between the layers, and making sure you add all the garlic. Cover with foil and bake in the oven for about $1^1/_2$ hours, until the potatoes are very tender.

5 Remove the foil, raise the heat a little, and bake for a further 10 to 15 minutes, until lightly browned on top.

Nutritional guidance
Per serving

477 calories
6 g protein
35 g fat (22 g saturated fat)
37 g carbohydrate
3 g fiber
91 mg sodium

✔✔   vitamin A
✔   vitamin C

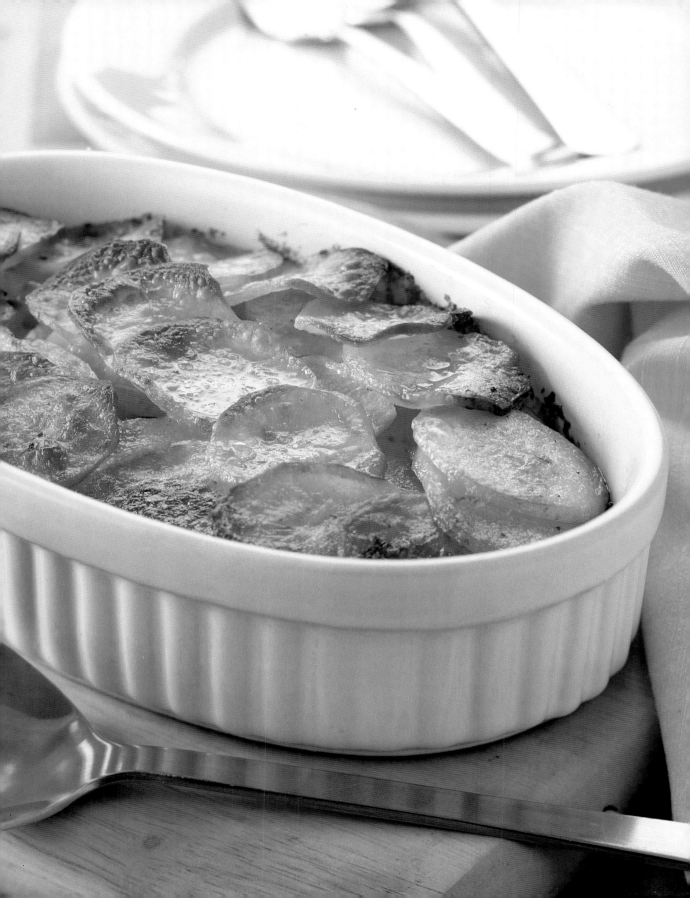

Soothing Rice

Pilaf

Serve this subtle, fragrant pilaf as an accompaniment to spicy dishes or even on its own when you want something to soothe a fragile stomach.

Serves 4 • Preparation time: 10 minutes • Cooking time: 20 minutes

1 tablespoon olive oil
1½ tablespoons butter
1 small onion, chopped fine
¾ cup basmati rice
1½ cups water or light chicken or vegetable broth

1 cinnamon stick, broken in half
2 cardamom pods, lightly cracked
1 bay leaf
1 heaping tablespoon golden raisins

1 heaping tablespoon slivered almonds
Salt and freshly ground black pepper

1 Heat the oil and 1 tablespoon of the butter in a heavy-based saucepan, add the onion, and cook gently until softened.

2 Add the rice and cook, stirring, for a couple of minutes, until it is coated in the oil and butter and has become opaque.

3 Add the water or broth, cinnamon, cardamom, bay leaf, and golden raisins. Bring to a boil, then cover with a tight-fitting lid, and cook over the lowest possible heat for 10 minutes, until the rice is just tender and the liquid has been absorbed.

4 Meanwhile, heat the remaining butter in a small skillet until sizzling, add the almonds, and fry until golden. Turn out onto a plate.

5 Once the rice is done, allow it to stand, covered, for 5 minutes, then fluff up with a fork and mix in the almonds.

Nutritional guidance
Per serving

264 calories
4 g protein
9 g fat (3 g saturated fat)
41 g carbohydrate
1 g fiber
40 mg sodium

✔ phosphorus, iron, vitamin E

Chinese Mixed Greens

with Oyster Sauce and Sesame Oil

Vegetables retain much of their nutrient content during stir-frying and absorb very little fat, so it's a good technique to try with any sort of greens, from spinach to kale, to Asian greens, such as these.

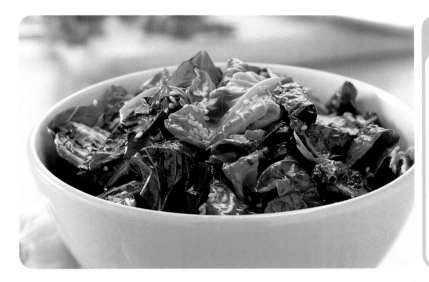

Nutritional guidance
Per serving

133 calories
7 g protein
8 g fat (1 g saturated fat)
9 g carbohydrate
7 g fiber
664 mg sodium

✔✔ calcium, iron,
    vitamin C,
    vitamin A
✔   folate,
    vitamin B12

Serves 2 • Preparation time: 15 minutes • Cooking time: 15 minutes

2 teaspoons peanut oil
2 teaspoons sesame oil
1 large clove garlic, chopped fine

¹/₄ teaspoon salt
14 ounces mixed greens, such as
   bok choy and Chinese cabbage,
   leaves torn up if large

2 tablespoons oyster sauce
¹/₄ teaspoon sesame seeds
   (optional)

1   Heat the peanut oil and 1 teaspoon of the sesame oil in a wok or large skillet, add the garlic and salt, and stir-fry over medium heat for 1 to 2 minutes, until the garlic is just beginning to color.

2   Add the bok choy and cabbage and stir-fry for 1 to 2 minutes, until just beginning to wilt, then add 1 tablespoon water, cover, and cook for 2 minutes. Uncover the skillet, raise the heat, and add the oyster sauce. Toss well and cook for 1 minute.

3   Stir in the remaining sesame oil, remove from the heat, sprinkle with sesame seeds if desired, and serve immediately.

Red Cabbage
with Apples and Raisins

A slow-cooked dish that tastes all the better for being prepared in advance and then reheated. It is good with lamb, pork, or game or, less conventionally, with a well-flavored cheese such as a mature goat cheese.

Serves 4 • Preparation time: 20 minutes • Cooking time: 50 minutes

1/4 stick butter
1 small onion, diced fine
1 clove garlic, minced
1 small red cabbage, cored and sliced into strips

1/4 cup soft brown sugar
6 tablespoons red wine vinegar
2/3 cup fresh apple juice (not from concentrate)
1/2 cinnamon stick

1/3 cup raisins
1 sweet, firm apple, cored and diced
Salt and freshly ground black pepper

1 Melt the butter in a heavy-based saucepan, add the onion and garlic, then cover and cook gently until softened.

2 Stir in the cabbage and cook for a few minutes until it is beginning to wilt. Stir in the sugar and red wine vinegar, raise the heat, and cook, stirring occasionally, until the cabbage looks slightly translucent.

3 Add the apple juice, cinnamon, raisins, and some salt and pepper and bring to a boil, then reduce the heat, cover, and cook gently for 30 minutes.

4 Stir in the diced apple and cook for a further 10 minutes or so, until tender. Taste and adjust the seasoning.

Nutritional guidance
Per serving

185 calories
2 g protein
6 g fat (3 g saturated fat)
33 g carbohydrate
4 g fiber
70 mg sodium

✔✔ vitamin C
✔ calcium, folate

Boston

Baked Beans

Canned baked beans are a useful standby to keep in the cupboard but once in a while it's worth making the real thing. They are as different from each other as white sliced bread and a homemade loaf. You can eat these beans as an accompaniment but they also make a meal served with crusty bread, mashed potatoes, or on toast. Omit the bacon if you want a vegetarian version.

Serves 8 • Preparation time: 25 minutes, plus soaking overnight • Cooking time: $3^1/_2$ hours

1 pound dried navy beans, soaked
  in cold water overnight
1 bay leaf
1 small onion, cut in half
5 ounces bacon, diced
1 large onion, diced fine

1 clove garlic, minced
$^1/_4$ cup soft dark brown sugar
2 tablespoons molasses
2 teaspoons dry mustard
$^1/_2$ cup puréed tomatoes
2 tablespoons ketchup

1 tablespoon Worcestershire
  sauce
Freshly ground black pepper

1 Drain the soaked beans then put them in a saucepan with the bay leaf and the halved onion, cover with plenty of fresh water, and bring to a boil. Boil hard for 10 minutes then reduce the heat and simmer until tender – about 40 minutes. Drain, reserving the cooking liquid, and set aside.

2 Preheat the oven to 325°F.

3 Fry the diced bacon in a large, heavy-based, ovenproof pot over a low heat until the fat begins to run. Add the diced onion and the garlic and fry until tender. Stir in the sugar and molasses then the mustard, puréed tomatoes, ketchup, Worcestershire sauce, and salt. Add the drained beans and season with plenty of black pepper, then stir in enough of the bean cooking liquid to cover everything.

3 Bring to a boil then cover and transfer to the oven to bake for $2^1/_2$ hours, stirring occasionally and topping up with water if the beans become too dry. If you need to reheat the beans before serving you can do this on top of the stove and you will probably need to add some water.

NOTE: Baked beans can be frozen, so it is worth making a large batch, like the quantity above.

Nutritional guidance
Per serving

269 calories
16 g protein
6 g fat (2 g saturated fat)
42 g carbohydrate
10 g fiber
489 mg sodium

✔   calcium,
    phosphorus, iron

Minted Peas
and Leeks

An easy way to add interest to frozen peas. Serve as an accompaniment to broiled or roasted chicken or fish.

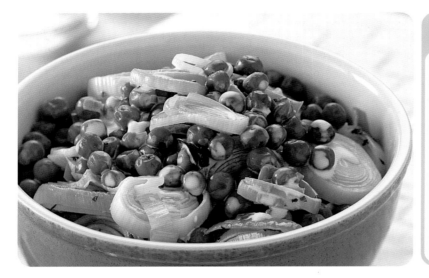

Nutritional guidance
Per serving

89 calories
5 g protein
5 g fat (3 g saturated fat)
8 g carbohydrate
4.5 g fiber
33 mg sodium

✔   vitamin A,
phosphorus, iron,
vitamin B, folate,
vitamin C

Serves 4 • Preparation time: 15 minutes • Cooking time: 15 minutes

1 tablespoon butter	Freshly grated nutmeg	1 to 2 tablespoons light cream
2 small leeks, white and light green parts sliced fine	2 teaspoons chopped mint 1 1/2 cups frozen peas	Salt and freshly ground black pepper

1   Melt the butter in a saucepan, add the leeks, then cover and cook gently until completely soft. Season with nutmeg, salt, and pepper and stir in the mint.

2   Cook the peas in boiling salted water, then drain.

3   Stir the peas into the leeks and then stir in enough light cream to bind the mixture loosely. Heat through gently and serve.

Cherry Tomatoes
sautéed with Basil

A quick accompaniment that makes a pleasant change from tomato salad, and is hardly any more effort to produce.

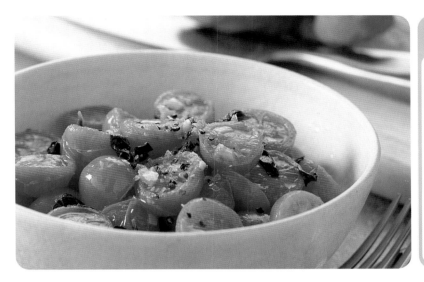

Nutritional guidance
Per serving

96 calories
1 g protein
8 g fat (2 g saturated fat)
5 g carbohydrate
1 g fiber
35 mg sodium

✔   vitamin A,
vitamin C,
vitamin E

Serves 2 • Preparation time: 5 minutes • Cooking time: 5 minutes

1 tablespoon olive oil
Small piece of butter
1 small clove garlic, minced

1½ cups cherry tomatoes, cut in half
Small pinch of sugar

About 5 basil leaves
Salt and freshly ground black pepper

1. Heat the olive oil and butter in a skillet until sizzling gently. Add the garlic, then the tomatoes, cut-side down. Cook gently for a minute or two, until the tomatoes are just beginning to soften, then turn them over and cook for another minute until heated through (be careful not to overcook them; they should retain their shape).

2. Sprinkle over the sugar and some salt and pepper, tear in the basil leaves, and stir well. Serve immediately.

Desserts, Cakes, and Cookies

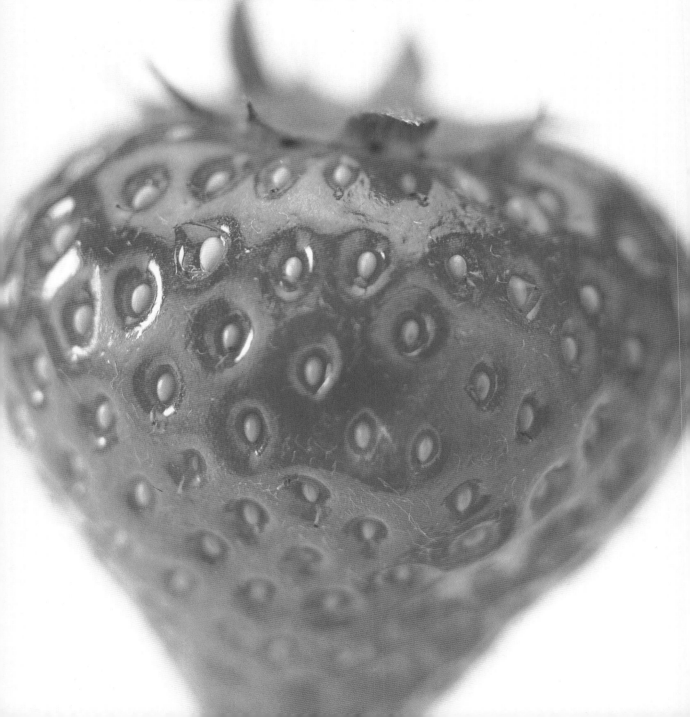

Light Lemon
Pudding

Also known as lemon surprise pudding, this is renowned for its magical ability to separate into two layers while cooking – a light lemon sponge with a thick custard underneath. It is good served with cream or fresh raspberries (or both).

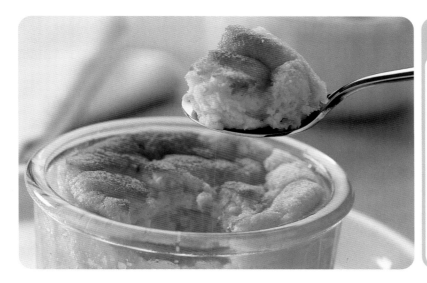

Nutritional guidance
Per serving

286 calories
7 g protein
15 g fat (8 g saturated fat)
33 g carbohydrate
0.4 g fiber
130 mg sodium

✔✔   vitamin B12
✔   calcium,
     phosphorus
     vitamin A

Serves 4 • Preparation time: 20 minutes • Cooking time: 40 minutes

$^1/_2$ stick unsalted butter
$^1/_3$ cup superfine sugar
Grated zest and juice of 1 large
    lemon

2 eggs, separated
$^1/_2$ cup all-purpose flour
$^3/_4$ teaspoon baking powder
$^1/_4$ teaspoon salt

1$^1/_4$ cups milk
Pinch of salt

1   Preheat the oven to 350°F.

2   Beat the butter, sugar, and lemon zest together until pale and fluffy. Beat in the egg yolks one at a time, then sift in the flour, baking powder, and salt, and mix in. Stir in the milk a little at a time, followed by the lemon juice. Don't worry if the mixture curdles.

3   In a separate bowl, whisk the egg whites with the salt until stiff. Fold them into the lemon mixture and pour into a greased 2$^1/_2$-pint ovenproof dish. Place in a roasting pan containing 1 inch hot water and bake for 30 to 40 minutes, until the top is golden brown and just firm to the touch. This is best served hot, although it's pretty good cold as well.

Blackberry and Apple

Strudel

Don't be daunted by the idea of making a strudel. Using filo pastry means that putting one together is a simple assembly job, with no special culinary skill required. Blackberries, or as an alternative, raspberries, make this strudel a particularly juicy one.

Serves 4 • Preparation time: 40 minutes • Cooking time: 30 minutes

1 cup fresh fine white bread crumbs

1 pound sweet, firm apples, peeled, cored, and sliced thin

Grated zest of $\frac{1}{2}$ lemon

2 tablespoons lemon juice

$\frac{1}{2}$ teaspoon ground cinnamon

3 tablespoons superfine sugar

$\frac{1}{2}$ cup roasted hazelnuts, chopped (optional)

$\frac{3}{4}$ cup blackberries, or raspberries

3 sheets filo pastry, about 16 x 18 inches

3 tablespoons unsalted butter, melted

1 heaping teaspoon confectioners' sugar

1 Preheat the oven to 375°F. Toast the bread crumbs in a large skillet over medium heat for about 5 minutes, stirring frequently, until lightly browned. Remove from the heat and set aside.

2 Put the sliced apples in a large bowl and mix with the lemon zest and juice, then add the cinnamon, sugar, hazelnuts, if using, and blackberries and mix together, being careful not to crush the blackberries.

3 Spread a clean dishtowel out on a work surface, place one of the sheets of filo pastry on it, and brush with some of the melted butter. Cover with another sheet of filo and brush with more butter, then top with the remaining sheet and brush with butter again. Sprinkle the browned bread crumbs over the pastry and then spread the apple and blackberry filling on top, leaving a good 1-inch border all the way round. Fold in the two short edges, then fold in the long edges. Starting at the long end nearest you, roll up the strudel, using the dishtowel to lift it slightly and making sure the ends stay folded in.

4 Transfer the strudel to a greased baking sheet, curving it gently into a horseshoe shape if necessary to fit (if the pastry tears at all, you can patch it with another sheet of filo). Brush with the remaining melted butter and bake in the oven for about 30 minutes, until golden brown.

5 Dust with the confectioners' sugar and serve warm, with cream or yogurt.

NOTE: The strudel can be frozen either before or after baking.

Nutritional guidance
Per serving

261 calories
4 g protein
9 g fat (5.5 g saturated fat)
43 g carbohydrate
4 g fiber
71 mg sodium

✔ vitamin A, vitamin C, vitamin E

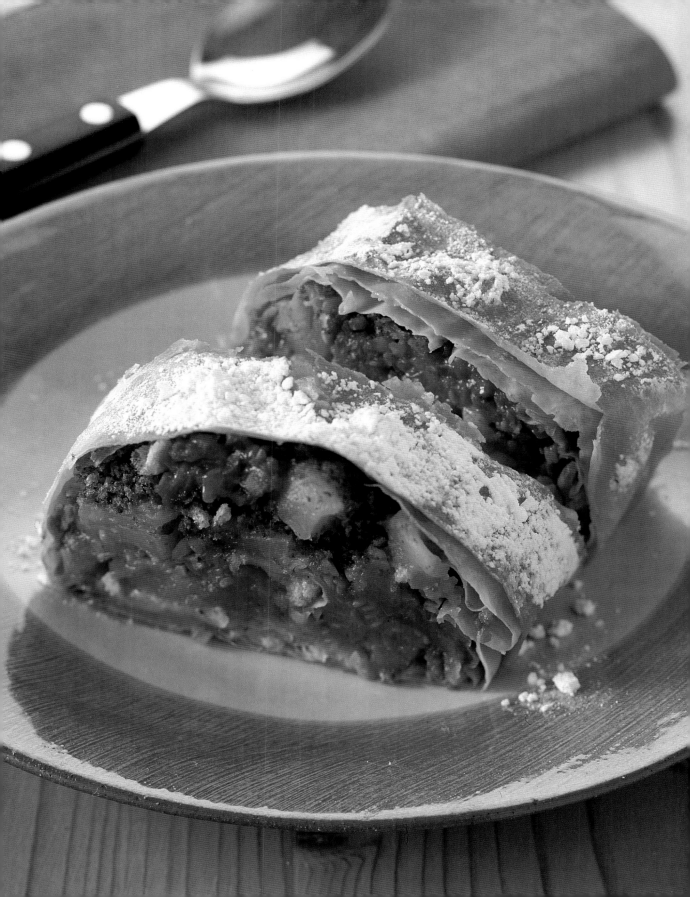

Mango Fool
with Hazelnut Cookies

Mangoes make a luscious, rich-tasting fool, so it's surprising to see how light the ingredients are here, with very little cream and only a couple of tablespoons of sugar. The cookies are more of an indulgence, but hazelnuts are good for you, being rich in essential fatty acids, among other things, so go ahead and indulge.

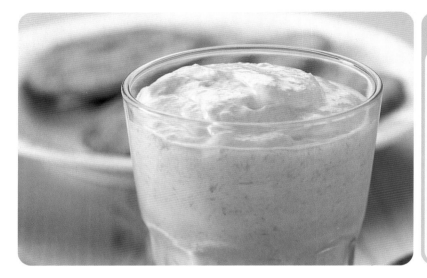

Nutritional guidance
Per serving

309 calories
5.5 g protein
18 g fat (11 g saturated fat)
34 g carbohydrate
2 g fiber
87 mg sodium

✔✔ vitamin A,
vitamin C
✔ calcium,
phosphorus,
vitamin E

Serves 2 • Preparation time: 25 minutes • Cooking time: 8 to 10 minutes

1 large very ripe mango
2 tablespoons confectioners'
   sugar

¹/₃ cup whipping cream
4 tablespoons yogurt
Squeeze of lemon juice (optional)

For the hazelnut cookies:
³/₄ cup roasted hazelnuts
¹/₃ cup superfine sugar
³/₄ cup all-purpose flour
³/₄ stick unsalted butter, diced

1 **To make the cookies:** process the hazelnuts in a food processor until coarsely ground. Add the sugar, flour, and butter and blend, until the mixture comes together to form a dough. Transfer to a piece of foil and shape into a short log, about 3 inches thick. Wrap in the foil and chill until firm.

2 **To make the fool:** peel the mango and cut the flesh from the pit, putting it in the cleaned food processor. Make sure you catch any juice. Add the confectioners' sugar and blend to a purée.

3 In a bowl, whip the cream until fairly stiff. Fold in the yogurt, followed by the mango purée. Taste and add a squeeze of lemon juice if desired. Pour into tall glasses and chill for at least 30 minutes.

4 Preheat the oven to 325°F. Cut thin slices from the cookie dough and place them on a baking sheet lined with baking parchment. Bake for 8 to 10 minutes, until lightly colored. Remove and allow to cool. Serve each portion of fool with two cookies.

NOTE: The recipe makes more cookies than you will need here; freeze the rest, or freeze the unbaked dough before slicing.

Baked Peaches
on Brioche

This simple way of serving fruit is equally good with pears or plums. If you have no brioche, use good-quality white bread instead.

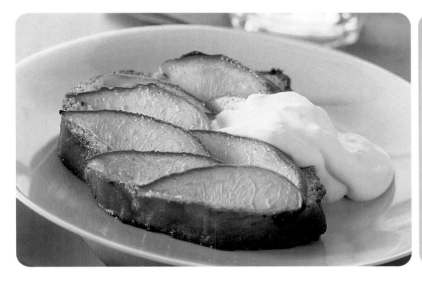

Nutritional guidance
Per serving

269 calories
3.5 g protein
11 g fat (5 g saturated fat)
42 g carbohydrate
2 g fiber
141 mg sodium

✔   vitamin A,
       phosphorus,
       vitamin C

Serves 4 • Preparation time: 10 minutes • Cooking time: 15 minutes

4 slices brioche, $^1/_2$ inch thick **Unsalted butter for spreading**	**4 tablespoons sugar, preferably** **vanilla sugar**	**2 large ripe peaches** **Juice of $^1/_2$ orange**

1   Preheat the oven to 400°F. Spread the brioche slices generously with butter, place on a baking sheet, and sprinkle evenly with about 3 tablespoons of the sugar.

2   Pit the peaches and slice thin, then put them in a bowl and mix with the orange juice. Arrange overlapping peach slices neatly on the brioche. Sprinkle with any orange juice left in the bowl, then with the remaining sugar.

3   Bake in an oven for about 15 minutes, until the brioche is crisp and golden and the peaches tender and lightly caramelized.

4   Serve immediately, with Greek yogurt if desired.

Sticky Almond Cake
with Summer Fruit Compote

This light cake has a lemon-flavored syrup poured over it to make it extra moist but it is almost as good without it if you prefer a plainer cake. Amaretti cookies are used instead of almond essence to give a subtle but distinctive flavor.

Serves 8 • Preparation time: 30 minutes • Cooking time: 1 hour

1½ sticks unsalted butter
⅔ cup superfine sugar
Grated zest of ½ lemon
3 eggs
¼ cup all-purpose flour
¾ cup ground almonds
½ cup amaretti cookies, crushed
   to fine crumbs

For the lemon syrup:
3 tablespoons superfine sugar
Juice of ½ large lemon

For the summer fruit compote:
4 ripe nectarines, pitted and
   sliced thin
⅔ cup blueberries
Juice of 1 orange

1   Preheat the oven to 350°F. Grease and line the bottom of a 7- inch springform cake pan, or 8-inch cake pan, with a round of waxed paper.

2   Beat the butter, sugar, and lemon zest together until pale and fluffy, then beat in the eggs one at a time, sifting in a little flour with each egg to prevent curdling. With a large metal spoon, fold in any remaining flour. Stir the ground almonds to remove any lumps, and then fold them into the mixture, followed by the amaretti crumbs.

3   Turn the mixture into the prepared cake pan and bake in the oven for about 1 hour, until the cake is risen, browned, and a skewer inserted into the center comes out just about clean (the cake should not be too dry). Remove from the oven and leave in the pan for 5 minutes.

4   Put the ingredients for the lemon syrup in a small saucepan and heat gently, stirring to dissolve the sugar. Remove the cake from its pan and place on a plate. Prick with a skewer a few times, and slowly spoon the syrup over the top so that it is absorbed into the warm cake. Allow to cool.

5   **To prepare the summer fruit compote:** Simply mix all the ingredients together and allow to marinate for about an hour. Serve with the cake.

NOTE: This cake can be frozen.

Nutritional guidance
Per serving

424 calories
7 g protein
27 g fat (13 g saturated fat)
41 g carbohydrate
2 g fiber
42 mg sodium

✔   vitamin A,
     phosphorus,
     vitamin C

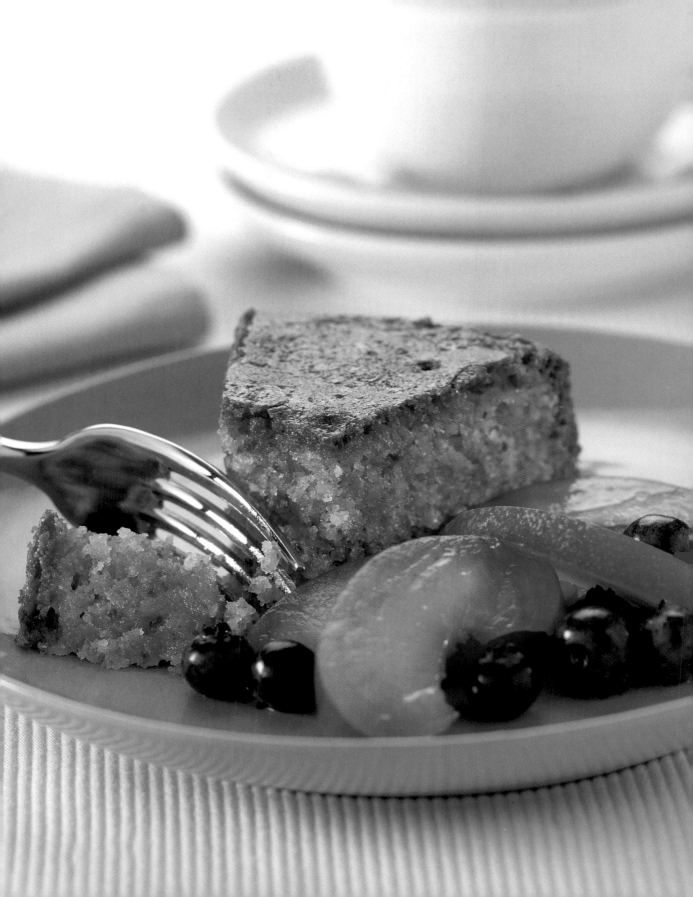

Peach and
Blueberry Crisp

A crisp is quicker to make than a pie, and is also lighter and easier to digest, with its simple topping. This recipe will adapt to all kinds of fruit which means you can use it year-round. Try apples instead of peaches or raspberries instead of blueberries.

Serves 4 • Preparation time: 20 minutes • Cooking time: 40 minutes

4 medium or 3 large ripe peaches, pitted and sliced
$1^1/_2$ cups blueberries
2 tablespoons superfine sugar
Fine grated zest of $^1/_2$ orange

For the topping:
$^3/_4$ cup all-purpose flour
Pinch each of ground cinnamon, nutmeg, and ground ginger
Pinch of salt
$^1/_4$ cup light brown sugar

$^3/_4$ stick unsalted butter, diced
$^1/_4$ cup toasted hazelnuts or almonds, chopped fine

1 Preheat the oven to 375°F.

2 In a bowl, toss the peaches with the blueberries, sugar, and orange zest and put them in a $2^1/_2$-pint baking dish.

3 **To prepare the topping:** Sift the flour, spices, and salt into a bowl and stir in the sugar. Rub in the butter with your fingertips until the mixture blends together. Stir in the nuts.

4 Scatter the topping mixture over the fruit and bake in the oven for about 40 minutes, until the topping is golden and crisp, and the juices are bubbling round the edges. Serve with cream, plain yogurt, or ice cream.

Nutritional guidance
Per serving

378 calories
4 g protein
20 g fat (10 g saturated fat)
49 g carbohydrate
3 g fiber
10 mg sodium

✔✔ vitamin A, vitamin C, vitamin E
✔ iron

Little Orange

Chocolate Pots

Classic chocolate mousse made with raw eggs is a forbidden treat during pregnancy but these little chocolate pots make a fine alternative when you feel in need of chocotherapy. They're easy to make, too, and are subtly flavored with orange.

Serves 4 • Preparation time: 15 minutes, plus chilling

4 ounces good-quality semisweet chocolate (at least 60% cocoa solids)

2 tablespoons orange juice
1 cup heavy cream
1 tablespoon superfine sugar
2 strips orange zest

A little whipping cream and some curls of orange zest, to decorate (optional)

1 Chop the chocolate quite fine with a large sharp knife and place in a bowl with the orange juice.

2 Put half the cream in a small pan with the sugar and strips of orange zest and bring to a boil very slowly, stirring occasionally to help dissolve the sugar. When it comes to a boil, remove from the heat and pour through a fine strainer onto the chocolate. Stir until the chocolate has melted, then set aside until just cool.

3 Whip the remaining cream until fairly stiff and fold into the chocolate mixture. Spoon into four ramekins and chill for at least 2 hours before serving.

4 Serve with some extra whipped cream, and orange zest curls on top for decoration.

NOTE: The chocolate pots can be frozen, although the orange flavor will fade slightly.

Nutritional guidance
Per serving

430 calories
2 g protein
37 g fat (23 g saturated fat)
23 g carbohydrate
1 g fiber
25 mg sodium

✔ vitamin A, phosphorus, vitamin E

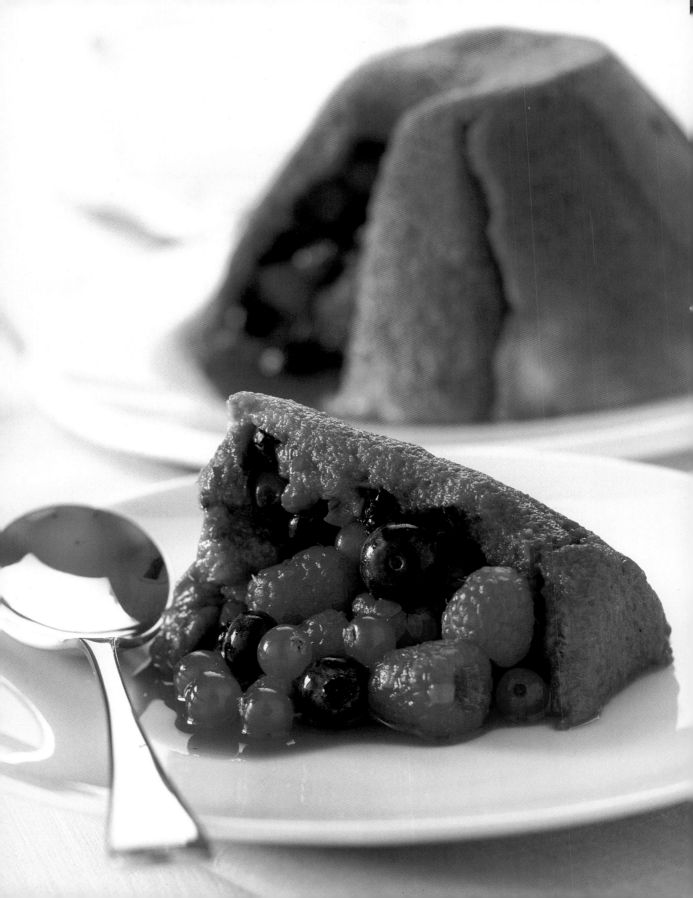

Summer Berry
Pudding

Summer pudding is remarkably good, full of intense fruit flavors. It is also a very healthy dessert, since it is absolutely bursting with vitamin C and contains virtually no fat. If red currants are not available, you can just increase the amount of raspberries by $^3/_4$ cup.

Serves 6 • Preparation time: 25 minutes • Cooking time: 3 minutes

2 cups raspberries	$^1/_2$ cup blueberries	About 8 slices good-quality white
$^3/_4$ cup red currants	$^1/_2$ cup superfine sugar	bread, cut about $^1/_2$ inch thick

1 Rinse all the fruit, then put it in a saucepan with the sugar and 2 tablespoons water. Place over gentle heat, bring just to a simmer, and cook for about 3 minutes, until the sugar has dissolved and there is lots of juice but the berries still hold their shape. Remove from the heat.

2 Cut off the crusts from the bread and cut a circle from one piece to fit the base of a 4-cup pudding mold, or soufflé dish. Cut the remaining slices diagonally in half and use them to line the sides of the mold, overlapping the slices and pressing them against the side of the bowl so they stay in place. If there are any gaps, cut pieces of bread to fit. Drizzle some of the juice from the fruit over the bread, then fill with the fruit and juice (there will probably be a little left; reserve this). Cut a final piece of bread to fit the top, so the fruit is completely enclosed. Cover with a plate that just fits inside the mold, then weigh it down (a couple of cans of tomatoes will do) and leave overnight in the refrigerator.

3 Shortly before serving, remove the weights and plate, and run a knife around the pudding to loosen the bread slightly from the mold. Put a plate on top and then, holding plate and mold together, invert it and give a slight shake. Remove the pudding mold; you should have an intact, but slightly wobbly pudding. If there are any pale patches of bread, pour over the reserved juice to color them.

4 Cut into wedges to serve – with cream, if desired.

NOTE: Summer pudding can be frozen in its pudding mold.

Nutritional guidance
Per serving

235 calories
6 g protein
1 g fat (0.3 g saturated fat)
53 g carbohydrate
4 g fiber
309 mg sodium

✔✔ vitamin C
✔ calcium, iron, folate

Figs

with Ricotta and Ginger

Always choose figs that feel heavy for their size and are so ripe they look as if they are about to burst.

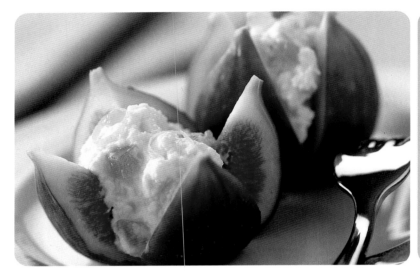

Nutritional guidance
Per serving

203 calories
9 g protein
9 g fat (5 g saturated fat)
25 g carbohydrate
2 g fiber
106 mg sodium

✔ calcium,
phosphorus,
vitamin A,
vitamin B12

Serves 2 • Preparation time: 5 minutes, plus chilling

²/₃ cup ricotta cheese
2 pieces candied ginger in syrup, diced fine

1 tablespoon syrup from the ginger jar, plus extra to drizzle

Grated zest of ¹/₂ lemon
4 large ripe figs

1 Mix together the ricotta cheese, ginger, syrup, and lemon zest and chill lightly.

2 Put the figs on serving plates, cut a deep cross in each one and open it up slightly. Fill with a generous spoonful of the ricotta mixture. Drizzle over a little extra syrup and serve.

Strawberry

Ice Cream

The great thing about this ice cream is that it doesn't contain eggs. It couldn't be simpler to make and has a pure, fresh flavor. Because this freezes much firmer than egg-based ice creams, remember to transfer it from the freezer to the refrigerator about an hour before serving to allow it to soften a little.

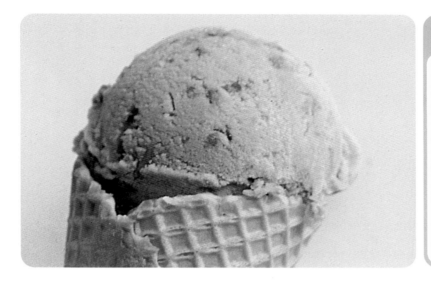

Nutritional guidance
Per serving

212 calories
2 g protein
12 g fat (8 g saturated fat)
25 g carbohydrate
1 g fiber
37 mg sodium

✔   vitamin C,
vitamin A,
calcium,
phosphorus

Serves 6 • Preparation time: 10 minutes, plus freezing

1 pound strawberries	Juice of ¹/₂ lemon	²/₃ cup low-fat yogurt
1 cup confectioners' sugar	²/₃ cup heavy cream	

1 Hull the strawberries and purée them in a food processor or blender with the confectioners' sugar and lemon juice.

2 In a bowl, whip the cream very lightly and fold in the yogurt, followed by the strawberry purée. Taste and add more lemon juice or sugar if necessary. Pour into a shallow bowl and place in the freezer until semifrozen.

3 Remove from the freezer and beat well with a fork or whisk, then taste it again, adjusting the balance of flavors if necessary. Freeze until firm.

Yogurt Cake
with Lemon Drizzle Glaze

Yogurt gives this cake a delicate pale crumb. If you don't feel like making the glaze, simply dust it with confectioners' sugar.

Serves 10 • Preparation time: 35 minutes • Cooking time: 40 minutes

3 large eggs, separated
2 tablespoons, plus
   1 cup superfine sugar
Grated zest of 1 lemon
³/₄ cup yogurt

³/₄ cup sunflower seed oil
2²/₃ cups all-purpose flour
1 tablespoon baking powder

For the lemon glaze:
³/₄ cup confectioners' sugar
3 to 4 teaspoons lemon juice

1   Preheat the oven to 325°F. Butter a 9-inch bundt pan and dust it lightly with superfine sugar.

2   Put the egg yolks, sugar, and lemon zest in a large mixing bowl and whisk together, preferably with an electric beater, until pale. Spoon the yogurt into a 2-cup measuring jug, top it up with the oil and then whisk the two into the egg mixture. Sift the flour and baking powder into the mixture and whisk briefly until combined.

3   In a separate bowl, whisk the egg whites until stiff then fold them gently into the mixture with a large metal spoon. Pour into the prepared pan and bake in the oven for about 40 minutes, until the cake is well risen and a skewer inserted in the center comes out clean. Leave in the pan for about 10 minutes, then loosen the edges with a knife and turn out onto a wire rack to cool.

4   **To prepare the lemon glaze:** Sift the confectioners' sugar into a bowl and gradually stir in enough lemon juice to make a glaze that runs slowly off the spoon. Drizzle it over the cake and allow to set.

NOTE: This cake can be frozen – preferably before you glaze it, or the glaze will soften it a little.

Nutritional guidance
Per serving

382 calories
6 g protein
17 g fat (2.5 g saturated fat)
54 g carbohydrate
1 g fiber
187 mg sodium

✔   calcium,
    phosphorus,
    vitamin E

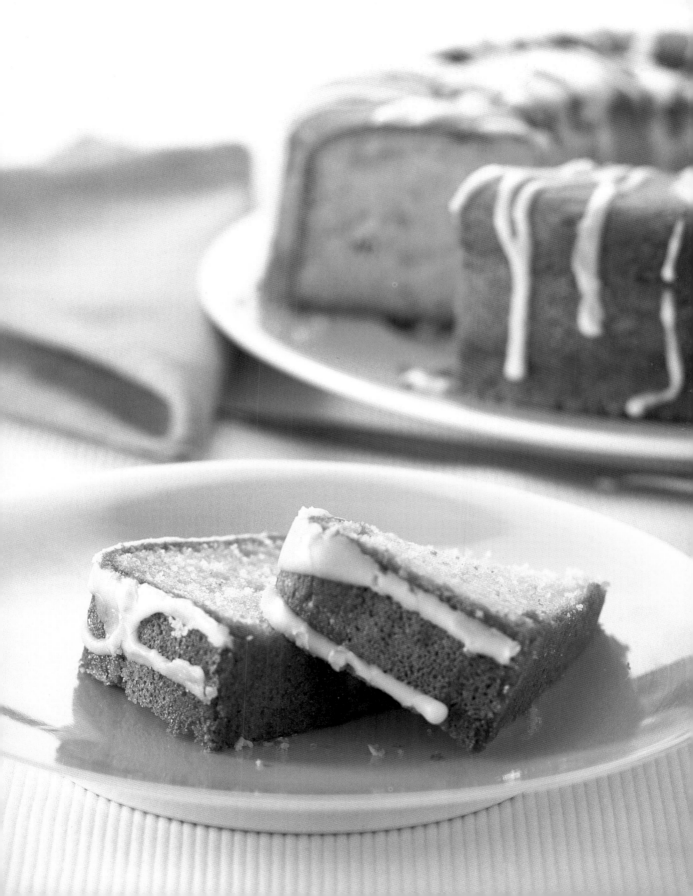

Prune and Golden Raisin

Teabread

Teabreads tend to be lower in fat than cakes but have a moist texture because the dry fruit is soaked in liquid before baking. This one is high in fiber and iron thanks to the prunes and tastes delicious. Enjoy it sliced and buttered for a snack or even for breakfast.

Makes a 2 pound loaf • Preparation time: 15 minutes, plus 2 hours soaking • Cooking time: about 1 hour

1 cup prunes, chopped
1/2 cup golden raisins
1/2 stick unsalted butter, diced
1 cup hot tea

2 cups self-rising flour
Pinch of salt
1/2 teaspoon pumpkin pie spice
1/2 cup light brown sugar

1 egg, lightly beaten

1 Preheat the oven to 350°F.

2 Put the prunes, golden raisins, and diced butter in a bowl. Pour over the hot tea, then cover and allow to stand for about 2 hours.

3 Sift the flour, salt, and spice into a bowl and stir in the sugar. Mix in the dry fruit and its soaking liquid then stir in the egg. The mixture should have a soft dropping consistency; if it is too stiff add a little milk or water.

3 Transfer the mixture to a greased 2-pound loaf pan and bake in the oven for about 1 hour, until it is well risen and a skewer inserted in the center comes out almost clean (the teabread should still be a little bit moist). Remove from the oven and leave in the pan for 10 minutes then turn out onto a wire rack to cool. The teabread can be eaten on the day it is made but improves with keeping. Wrap in foil and store in an airtight container.

NOTE: This teabread can be frozen. You could slice it before freezing then take out only as much as you need.

Nutritional guidance
Per serving

2075 calories
36 g protein
52 g fat (29 g saturated fat)
391 g carbohydrate
18.5 g fiber
136 mg sodium

✔ vitamin A, iron

Apricot and Sunflower Seed

Oat Bars

I've never come across anyone who doesn't love these oat bars. Although they can be quite high in fat and sugar, the good news is that the fiber in the oats helps to lower blood cholesterol levels and also slows the absorption of the sugar by your body. These bars have extra fiber – and extra flavor – from the dried apricots and sunflower seeds.

Makes 16 • Preparation time: 10 minutes • Cooking time: 20 to 25 minutes

1$^1/_4$ sticks butter
$^1/_3$ cup raw brown sugar
4 tablespoons corn syrup
2$^1/_4$ cups rolled oats

2 tablespoons sunflower seeds
$^1/_2$ cup dried apricots, chopped
Squeeze of lemon juice
Pinch of salt

1 Preheat the oven to 375°F. Grease an 8 or 9-inch square baking pan.

2 Put the butter, sugar, and corn syrup in a large saucepan and melt over a low heat, stirring occasionally. Remove from the heat, add all the remaining ingredients and stir well.

2 Turn into the baking pan and bake for 20 to 25 minutes, until turning brown around the edges. Do not overcook; the mixture will firm up as it cools. Leave until warm then mark into bars with a knife.

3 Cut into bars when cold and store in an airtight container.

NOTE: If the dried apricots are very dry, soak them first in hot water for 10 minutes to soften them. Drain before adding to the syrup mixture.
The oat bars can be frozen.

Nutritional guidance
Per serving

176 calories
2 g protein
10 g fat (5.5 g saturated fat)
21 g carbohydrate
1.5 g fiber
92 mg sodium

✔ vitamin A,
vitamin B1,
vitamin E

Triple-ginger
Cookies

If ginger is your number-one weapon in the war against morning sickness, try these cookies. They contain ground and candied ginger as well as gingerroot, giving them a subtle, spicy heat and great anti-nausea properties.

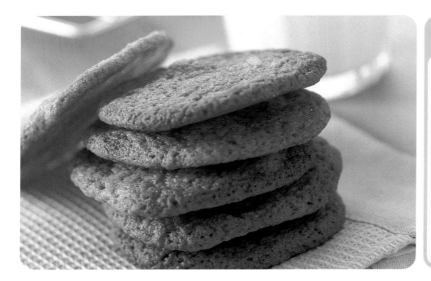

Nutritional guidance
Per serving

73 calories
1 g protein
2 g fat (1 g saturated fat)
13 g carbohydrate
0.3 g fiber
62 mg sodium

✔ vitamin A,
vitamin E

Makes about 30 • Preparation time: 10 minutes • Cooking time: 10 to 12 minutes

¹/₂ cup corn syrup	3 pieces candied ginger, diced fine	1 teaspoon ground ginger
³/₄ stick unsalted butter, diced	2 cups self-rising flour	Pinch of salt
1-inch piece gingerroot, grated		¹/₂ cup superfine sugar
		1 egg, lightly beaten

1 Preheat the oven to 325°F. Spray the inside of a measuring cup with cooking spray before pouring in the corn syrup. This will help prevent the syrup sticking to the cup, making it easier to remove. Pour the corn syrup into a small pan. Add the butter and then place the pan over low heat, stirring occasionally until the butter has melted. Remove from the heat and stir in the gingerroot and candied ginger.

2 Sift the flour, ground ginger, and salt into a bowl and stir in the sugar. Pour in the melted mixture and mix well with a wooden spoon, then add the egg and mix until smooth.

3 Spoon teaspoonfuls of the cookie mixture on a cookie sheet lined with baking parchment, spacing them about 3 inches apart (cookies will spread).

4 Bake in the oven, in batches, allowing about 10 minutes for slightly soft cookies or a couple of minutes longer for crisper ones. Transfer to a wire rack to cool.

NOTE: These cookies can be frozen.

Caraway

Cookies

Caraway seeds are said to increase the milk flow in breastfeeding mothers. It sounds like a good excuse for stocking up on these cookies ready for after your baby is born. They are also good to nibble if you are feeling queasy because they have a crumbly, slightly dry texture, and are not too sweet. If you do not care for the taste of caraway, either omit the seeds, or replace them with $1/2$ teaspoon ground cinnamon and/or 2 tablespoons currants.

Makes about 20 • Preparation time: 15 minutes • Cooking time: 12 to 15 minutes

2 cups self-rising flour
$1/2$ cup superfine sugar

1 stick unsalted butter, diced
Grated zest of $1/2$ lemon
1 teaspoon caraway seeds

1 egg, lightly beaten
1 to 2 teaspoons lemon juice

1 Preheat the oven to 350°F.

2 Sift the flour into a bowl, stir in the sugar, then rub in the butter with your fingertips until the mixture resembles fine crumbs. Stir in the lemon zest and caraway seeds then add the egg and enough lemon juice to form a soft but not sticky dough.

3 Put heaping teaspoons of the mixture on a cookie sheet lined with baking parchment, spacing them about 3 inches apart (you will have to cook them in batches). Press each one down lightly with the back of a fork – dust it with flour if it sticks.

4 Bake the cookies in the oven for 12 to 15 minutes, until lightly colored, then transfer to a wire rack to cool.

NOTE: These cookies can be frozen.

Nutritional guidance
Per serving

98 calories
1 g protein
5 g fat (3 g saturated fat)
14 g carbohydrate
0.4 g fiber
46 mg sodium

✔ vitamin A, phosphorus

Whole-wheat Currant

Scones

These scones are only lightly sweetened and are a wholesome way to keep hunger pangs at bay. Scones freeze well, so make extra to store in the freezer ready for after your baby is born.

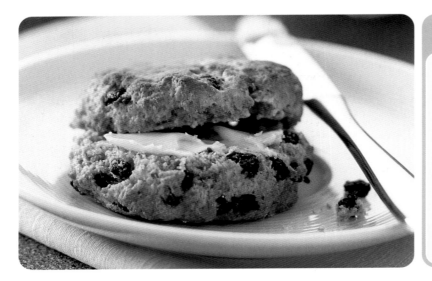

Nutritional guidance
Per serving

182 calories
5 g protein
6 g fat (3 g saturated fat)
30 g carbohydrate
2 g fiber
197 mg sodium

✔ vitamin A, phosphorus

Makes 8 • Preparation time: 20 minutes • Cooking time: 12 minutes

1¹/₂ cups whole-wheat flour
¹/₂ cup all-purpose flour
1 tablespoon baking powder
Pinch of salt

3 tablespoons superfine sugar
3 tablespoons unsalted butter, diced
¹/₂ cup currants

1 egg
¹/₃ cup milk

1   Preheat the oven to 425°F. Sift the flours, baking powder, and salt into a bowl and stir in the sugar. Rub in the butter with your fingertips until the mixture resembles fine crumbs then stir in the currants.

2   Lightly whisk the egg and milk together, then pour into the mixture and stir together with a round-bladed knife until it forms a soft but not sticky dough; you might not need all the liquid, so hold a little back.

3   Turn out onto a floured board and pat out to about 1 inch thick (the scones rise better if you fold the dough over a couple of times while doing this). Cut into rounds with a 2¹/₂- inch cookie cutter and place on a greased baking sheet. Press the trimmings together and reroll them to make more scones.

4   Brush the tops with any leftover egg and milk, or with a little extra milk, and bake in the oven for about 12 minutes, until risen and golden. Transfer to a wire rack and allow to cool.

NOTE: The scones can be frozen.